The
Little Book of
Big
Life Change

A Nine-Part Journey to Feeling
WHOLE

CARRIE CIULA

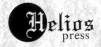

Helios Press books may be purchased in bulk at special discounts for sales promotion, corporate gifts, fund-raising, or educational purposes. Special editions can also be created to specifications. For details, contact the Special Sales Department, Skyhorse Publishing, 307 West 36th Street, 11th Floor, New York, NY 10018 or info@skyhorsepublishing.com.

Helios® and Helios Press® are registered trademarks of Skyhorse Publishing, Inc.®, a Delaware corporation.

Visit our website at www.skyhorsepublishing.com.

10 9 8 7 6 5 4 3 2 1

Library of Congress Cataloging-in-Publication Data is available on file.

Cover design by Laura Klynstra
Cover illustration by gettyimages

Hardcover ISBN: 978-1-5107-4716-6
Ebook ISBN: 978-1-5107-4719-7

Printed in China

To our knowing that we are never separate from the greatest love, the most beautiful truths, and the magic that is within and all around us.

Table of Contents

Foreword

I t can be all too easy to view the components of ourselves and of the world as separate, distinct, and autonomous. Too often, our inner world and outer world are not in full alignment; what our intuition tells us and what our brains tell us are juxtaposed. What we think we *should* do and what we *feel* are often different. This separation is at the core of the human condition. From this duality, all the other separateness arises. However, in the right light, it's possible to capture that it is all connected. The parts, the people, the processes. The interconnectedness of all things. Some of us have caught a glimpse of that utter connectedness in a moment of crisis or a moment of triumph. Some of us regularly touch it through a practice like meditation or exercise. But many of us spend too much time being separated from that whole state. Writer Anaïs Nin articulated, "We don't see the world as it is, we see it as we are." As true of an observance as true can be, it is the simple act and art of looking through a lens of wholeness that reveals the wholeness and interconnectedness of the world.

The Little Book of Big Life Change brings a breath of freshness, space, and connectedness in a time on the planet that can feel fractured, frenetic, and falling apart. This book shows us that whole-ness is as much of a practice as it is a process and that it is more than the sum of its parts. While wholeness may be more aptly called whole-*ish* in this day and age, this book will help you find yourself, where you are, tools and map in hand. In this book, Carrie shares the spirit of what feels like the magical art of tidying up our inner world to cultivate wholeness. She creates a framework to simplify complex topics into bite-size components and steps, from food guides and how to approach eating to herbal infusions and breathing practices; from joyful, physical movement to supporting rest naturally; from the power of positive thought and forgiveness to connecting to com-munity, ourselves, and the Earth. These pleasurable pages provide a practical map to integrate the components of our body, mind, and spirit to a balance that feels more and more and more whole.

—*Renée Loux,*
plant-based chef, four-time author, educator, researcher, journalist,
and natural products entrepreneur (visit her at reneeloux.com)

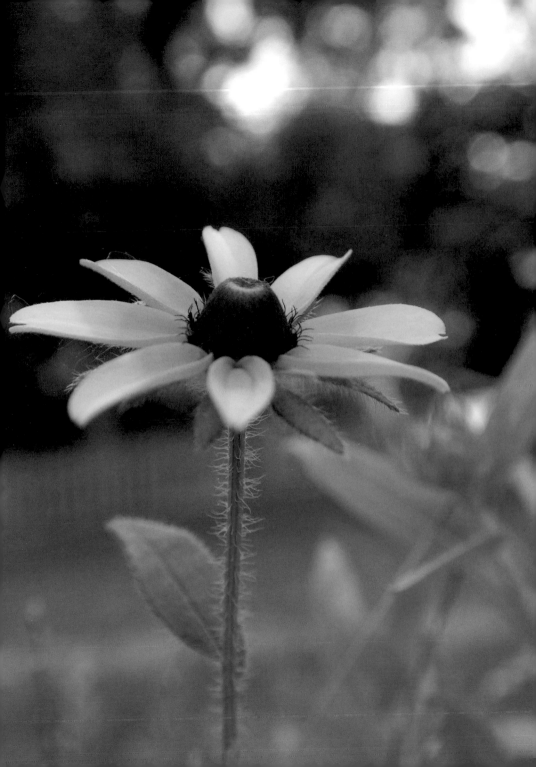

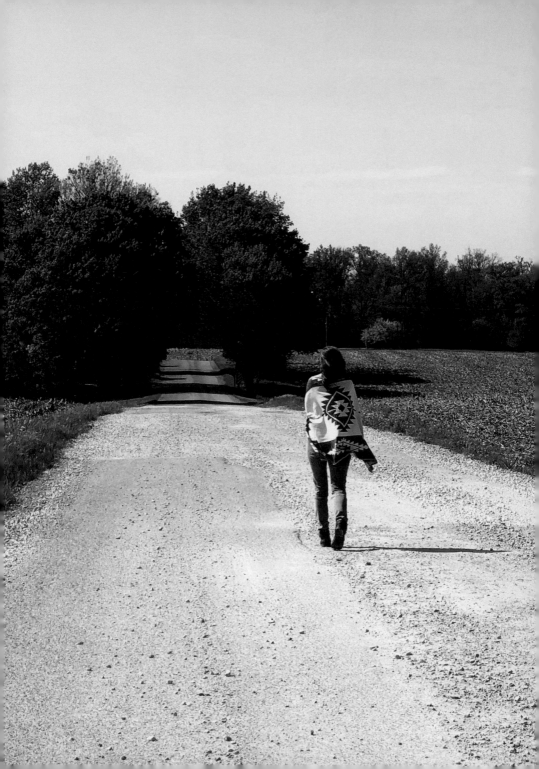

Introduction

I adore the way that hindsight often reveals perfection along our path. Most of us, even with our finest imaginative skills, would never be able to come up with the future string of events tying this very moment in our life to a random moment a handful of years down the road—yet when we look back, there seems to be a divine and resolute integration in the way things play out. We're all coming though this life with certain things that we are here to learn and to accomplish. What would your life look like if you could create it in a way that makes you feel most happy and whole? This is a question I love asking others. I've learned a lot from their responses—but first, a few steps into my own life-reframing story.

From a very young age, I recognized writing as something I really enjoy. By my college years, I was also shaping up to be a strong advocate for living in a more balanced and harmonious way with the natural world around us. After changing my major several times, I finally decided that I should be on track to working a nine-to-five salaried job. I interlaced my love for our Earth by choosing to learn how to teach biology and environmental science at the secondary level. I've always been intuitive, and I knew that I was making this choice through my mind alone. My heart and soul were never as accepting or as comfortably on board. Being off of my life path as it related to my career was, from the start, stressful. I finished school. I accepted a job in a town a little over an hour away from where I was living at the time. And, probably being too prepared, I channeled every bit of my thought, time, and energy into my work.

Sometimes, an awareness of a need for change becomes both apparent and accepted slowly over a stretch of time. Other times, it is wrapped up in a quick, pivotal moment. I experienced one of these unexpected, determining moments while in the computer lab with my 5th period environmental science class. Students were researching a pressing environmental issue when one of the quieter boys in the class out of seemingly nowhere walked up to me and began telling me how much he enjoyed the projects we were working on that year. He wrapped up by asking me if I was happy teaching. My spoken reply didn't match the reply that instantly formed in my core: *I wasn't.* I suddenly felt simultaneously embarrassed and regretful that I had put so much time into a career that I knew wasn't the best fit for me. I have no idea what he was thinking of when he asked me that particular question on that particular day, but it was a powerful universal nudge, and regardless of from whom or where or how it was presented to me, I am grateful for it. Less of a question, really, and more of an able pair of hands, his brief and piercing inquiry spun the entirety of my weight around and gently placed me on an entirely new course. I turned in my resignation letter a couple of weeks later.

By the end of that school year, I had traveled so far away from many of the things and activities I was most connected with and passionate about that I felt lost and exhausted. My journey to regain my own mind-body-spirit balance began, but my healing work with others didn't really take hold until one of our feline friends developed a condition that a local vet claimed he wouldn't survive. Uneager to take his heavy medication-strewn advice, I felt crucially hopeful for guidance outside of the allopathic community. One late, stormy night, I walked down to a pond near our home. I collapsed on the ground and began to weep. I had no idea who I was talking with or asking guidance from, but I knew that I wasn't alone, and I knew that I was fully surrendered and open to whatever came next. The days and weeks that followed repeatedly leave me without words, yet the foundation of what I took from this stretch is that the limits to what we believe is possible could use a little rethinking. Our cat's presence completely and lastingly shifted within days. This experience deepened my awareness of the ways that energy makes up and influences our physical world and unexpectedly commenced an intimate connection with spiritually and intuitively guided healing.

Change-starters. We all occasionally experience them. Moments and experiences that reframe the picture of our lives—that reorganize boundaries, that invite us to look at things in a different way and fine-tune our focus. Trailing my own change-starters, I spent some time simply sitting with and acclimating to both small and large shifts within and around my life and myself. At times, I felt unsettled for having traveled down certain paths. I also felt vulnerable, raw, trusting, and sincere with only the intention of *being*—unaware and unconcerned of any outcome—and a deep sense and knowing that, for a while, I was to be still, encircled by spiritual guidance. Slowly, my focus opened up from this stretch of just being to include a blended, potent combination of envisioning the life that I wanted to experience, knowing that this vision was possible, allowing divinely timed doors to open, and doing the work that was needed to pull this vision into my reality.

What I've stumbled upon over and over throughout the years is that wellness doesn't come from a bottle or a cleanse—it comes from being connected, from freely allowing and following fluent tides of passion, from making gut-based decisions, from indulging in openness, love, and authenticity—*always, in all ways*. I often shed a few grateful tears when I pause to think about how, if given the choice today, I wouldn't trade in any of this experience. Sometimes it takes a while, for each of us within our own unique life plans, to truly feel this. For all of our experiences, good and sometimes seemingly not so good, we can choose to feel grateful. This is an adventure—a beautiful, ongoing exploration—and there are pushes in our lives that allow each of us to reach the place where we are, as well as to be on the best-fit path to where we're going. I enjoy reading about and listening to stories from those coming through this life with the purpose of healing, and I've noticed that many of these people have one thing in common: they've experienced challenging events or situations that have placed them, out of necessity, in the direction of a more wholly immersed understanding. It makes sense, doesn't it? What deeper-rooted or more significant way to learn about how to help others than to first learn how to help one's self?

Again, what would your life look like if you could create it in a way that makes you feel most happy and whole? It feels like such an important question, and what I've learned through asking it is that most people have an immediate and pretty clear idea about the life that would best support them feeling well. While sifting through all of the uncertain, quickly changing information and culturally directed notions about what our lives should look like, this idea often becomes less clear. I've learned that when we tune in to a few timelessly effective elements of feeling whole, as well as our own wise internal voice, we already have a lot of the answers that we seem to be constantly searching for.

This project represents the culmination of several years of boundless research, of trials, of settling into myself, of working with others, and of soulful evolution—collectively, of life experience. I carry with me an insatiable curiosity around how we grew to place so much trust in present-day, business-centered pillars and paradigms of health and, likewise, how we can get back to living vibrant and intuitively guided lives. *The Little Book of Big Life Change* is, in essence, the distillation of these years of study and experience in the areas of nutrition, breath, movement, rest, cleansing, thought, unity, purpose, and love into a purposefully brief, manageable organization of these important areas of balance and well-being. Combining the mantra "I Am" with these nine essentials brews up a mixture of powerful affirmations with big life-reframing potential. I repeatedly witness the ways in which these affirmations help to guide and change lives. They gently lead us toward a deeper knowing that true balance happens as we learn to support the feeling of being content, connected, and complete within one's self—the feeling of being *whole*.

While the book you hold is a recent formation, the universal foundation is as old as the beginning of life. My intention is simply to remind us all about the basics of connection, love, and health that seem to have been lost, forgotten, or misinterpreted as we began trading in passed down and/or innate understanding for the information sold by various government agencies, pharmaceutical companies, agricultural giants—even the know-it-all, multilevel marketer next door. Throughout this nine-part journey, you will find perennially effective information that was as relevant a hundred years ago as it will be a hundred years from now—information gifted to us from our surrounding world, if we choose to quiet our minds and to listen. You will find an authentic desire to contribute to the massive change that is taking place on our planet, and a deep understanding that supporting wholeness in others supports wholeness in one's self and that, likewise, supporting wholeness in one's self supports wholeness in others and our world. We are cocreating change within and around us—personal *and* global change.

It is my hope and intention that you succeed in the dreams and goals that you envision. To be a small part of the process through passing along any information that might support your travel fills and sustains me—it is where and how I find a lot of my own happiness and wholeness. If you want to step a little farther along a path that makes you feel more balanced, I wrote this for you. If you want to step a lot farther and really shake things up, I wrote this for you. Wherever you're at and wherever you want to go, I invite you to settle in with this time-honored wisdom, to allow yourself to be inspired to incorporate some or all of it into your everyday life, and to be ready for lasting change.

To and for *this* journey,
—*ours*—
the deepest love and gratitude.

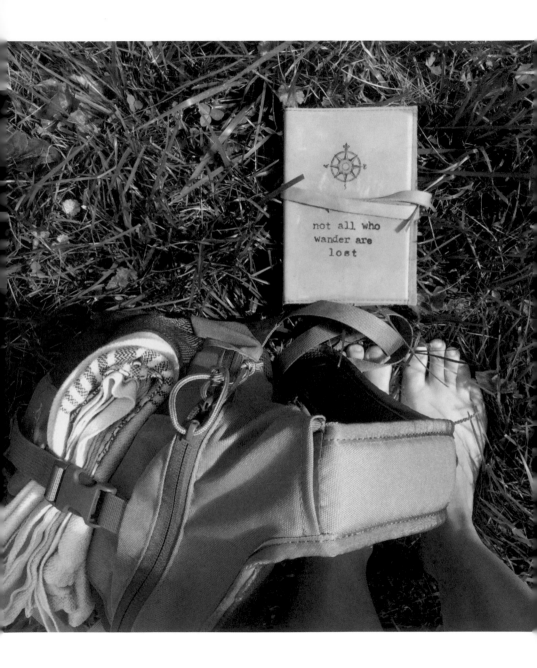

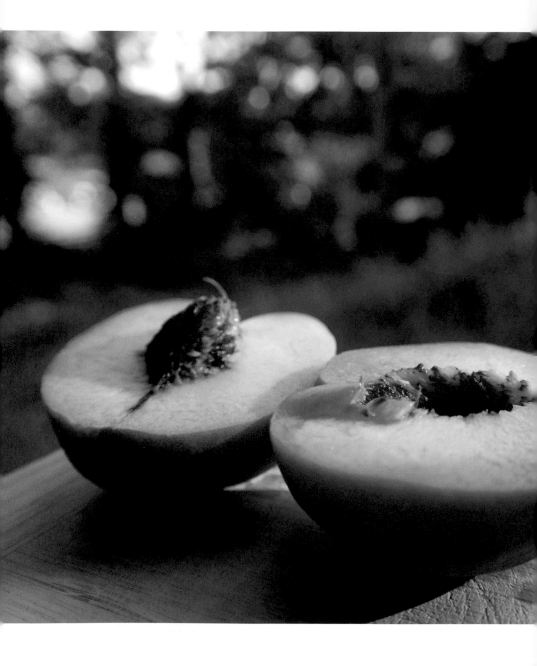

1

I Am Nourished (Nutrition)

🌿✨

"The wonderful thing about food is you get three votes a day.
Every one of them has the potential to change the world."
—Michael Pollan, author, journalist, and activist

Food is medicine in a way that goes far deeper than its obvious nutritional offerings. It holds a profound power throughout so many aspects of our lives. For many, the day begins and ends in the kitchen. Food and food preparation can be a primal foundation, with a pulse all its own, from which so many things are configured and shaped: how we feel, how we create, how we evolve—*how we connect*. We tend to underestimate the impact food has upon our lives and upon the world around us.

Years ago, after the decision to eliminate processed foods from my diet, I met with reactions that ran from genuine fear to playful teasing. When asked to describe a typical day's fare during that time of dietary transition, I would often hear a variation of the response "I'll just stick with a normal diet." The word "normal" amuses me. Today, in "normal America," we reside in a culture that perceives processed, manufactured foods as completely fine, yet a person who opts for fresh fare is viewed as socially defunct—somewhat of an extremist. Consider the "normal" journey of a grain of wheat; first, it is stripped of its fiber, healthy oils, vitamins, and minerals—virtually all of the nutrition it has to offer—then ground into flour, bleached with chemicals, and stamped into crackers, cereal, biscuits, pastries, and pasta. Once we begin looking at, really scrutinizing, the labels of *everything* we put into our mouths, the decision to eat whole foods becomes an easy one. Everything from soups to condiments (foods that are often touted as being "healthy") is filled with hydrogenated oils, high fructose corn syrup, chemicals, and preservatives that would never be acceptable if they weren't disguised in a can of fruit or a granola bar. When did it become "normal" for food companies to override nature in deciding what our bodies can and should use as fuel? And, more important, what *is* biologically normal?

While we have largely fallen out of the circle of passed down, slow-food tradition and inner knowing, thriving cultures around the world reveal one overriding dietary theme: they eat whole foods in Earth-provided form. These foods include an abundant variety of fresh fruits, land, sea, and root vegetables, leafy greens, soaked and sprouted nuts, seeds—and smaller amounts of insects, wild-caught fish, and animal-sourced products from clean, healthy, happy, *humanely, conscientiously raised* or wild animals. (Note: There is a lot of debate around whether humans are designed to eat certain animal products and/or grains. These food sources aside, many people thrive when they include plenty of fresh fruits, leafy greens, and vegetables in their daily fare. It is a personal choice whether to incorporate animal products and/or grains into one's life and diet; and this choice can, in part, be based on individual biomolecular compositions, constitutions, genetic lineage, or intuition. Keep in mind how important it is, when choosing animal products, to buy and support humanely raised or wild animals and to entirely avoid the whole spectrum of factory-farmed products lining conventional store shelves. Also consider, despite their being the foundation of the food pyramid that many of us grew up learning about, that grains might not be a good dietary fit for every person—especially the genetically modified, highly processed grain-strewn foods that currently line market shelves. If you are experiencing any type of digestive issues, this topic is worth further researching.)

During my own self-directed quest, I have tried countless whole foods based ways of eating. I have eaten vegetarian and vegan fare. I discovered the benefits of raw foods and ate uncooked meals for seven years. I have practiced Body Ecology principles, incorporated the wisdom of Ayurveda into our meal making, explored macrobiotics, experimented with the blood-type theory, studied the work of Weston Price, and have appreciated a paleo way of eating. I love to forage for and eat wild food and, along this entire path, have blended up hundreds of green smoothies. While all of these approaches and paradigms have had things to offer, none have come into my life waving around a golden ticket. There is no sweeping, absolute health or dietary strategy that will work the same for every person. Things shift. People are different and always changing. I really enjoy what I've been able to learn from my experiences with various ways of eating, and there are bits and pieces that I have incorporated into my life from each, yet the ways of eating (and of living) that I consistently come back to and am most comfortable with are intuitive and constantly adapting to both personal and environmental factors.

Five Foundational Nourishment Guidelines

Though I don't adhere to a one-size-fits-all approach, I love to simplify what can feel like a complex issue by focusing on five foundational nourishment guidelines. These guidelines are powerful. For us all, they have the ability to create big change!

1. **Eat fresh and whole** (mostly organic, heirloom, local, wild, entirely real, Earth-made) **foods.**
2. **Eat simple food combinations.**
3. **Avoid overeating and nighttime eating.**
4. **Allow your intuition to be your guide.**
5. **Nourish intentionally with the spirit of love and gratitude.**

Eat Fresh and Whole Foods

The study of nutritional science is increasingly complex and easily misrepresented and misunderstood. Our current culture tends to want to pick apart and isolate the function of many things. However, understanding the needs of complex orchestrations, such as our ecosystem and our bodies, gets complicated very quickly. In any ecosystem, removing just one seemingly insignificant population or species will often result in far-reaching shifts for the entire community. In our bodies, removing certain nutrients can have this same unbalancing effect. Certain nutrients require certain factors to be put to use;

some minerals need others in order to be absorbed effectively; particular vitamins double as coenzymes to help other vitamins work properly. For example, adequate amounts of vitamins A, D, and K2 are needed for calcium absorption and placement. Vitamin C aids in the absorption of iron and has the ability to regenerate supplies of vitamin E. The further we take this all apart, the deeper the connections go—which is why the hottest trends in the diet and nutrition world are always changing. So, how can we ensure that we're receiving the nutrients our bodies require? By focusing on a diet rich in fresh, whole foods that have been grown in rich, healthy soil.

Whole foods are a complete package. Foods, in the form that our Earth created them, retain much of their original nutritional value. These foods have not been stripped of nutrients by high-tech machinery; polluted with artificial ingredients, additives, colorings, or preservatives; smashed and packaged into "convenient" (often wasteful) containers; transported on conveyor belts; shipped across the country; and strategically placed on market shelves, where they could sit for months, if not years, awaiting their consumption. Processed, isolated, denatured, packaged-for-the-long-haul creations are difficult for the body to recognize and therefore translate into anything useful. On the flip side, our bodies immediately recognize the nutritional offerings of whole foods and know how to use them effectively. Fresh, whole foods offer an entirely different experience. They *feel* different. They are lush, vibrant, full of subtle and not-so-subtle flavors, and *contain the nutrients that our bodies need in the form and balance that our bodies need them in.* Our life and presence mirror our fuel. When we consume food that is clean, colorful, and full of vitality and life force, we build and sustain a presence that is more whole, balanced, colorful, and full of this transferred vitality and life force.

—Foods to Avoid—

These foods deplete the body of vital nutrients and energy. They are best avoided for optimal health.

- All refined sugars
- Processed and packaged foods including crackers, chips, and boxed cereals
- Baked goods (breads, muffins, cakes, cookies, etc.)
- Margarine or other alternatives to butter
- Canned/jarred foods (soups, sauces, and condiments with lengthy lists of ingredients)
- Artificial sweeteners
- Soda and bottled (high sugar) juices
- Fast foods and chain restaurant foods
- Processed factory meat (hot dogs, lunch meat, both ground and whole cuts)
- Mass-produced, homogenized, pasteurized dairy
- Mass-produced eggs from non-grass-fed hens

—Foods to Enjoy—

These nutrient-dense, clean-energy foods promote optimal health and cellular function. Aside from eating biologically appropriate, real food, there are no set guidelines for good nutrition. We can each learn what works for us—vary our meals, increase our amount of wild and live foods, and enjoy what we choose to eat. Ideally, the following foods should be locally and organically grown.

- Leafy greens and herbs (chard, kale, spinach, cilantro, dill, etc.)

- Lettuces (red leaf, green leaf, Boston, romaine, etc.)
- Wild greens (dandelion, wild spinach, chickweed, wild lettuce, purslane, etc.)
- Land veggies (broccoli, cauliflower, radishes, onions, etc.)
- Sea veggies (dulse, kelp, arame, wakame, etc.)

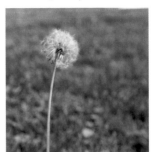

- Sprouts (red clover, alfalfa, sunflower, broccoli, etc.)
- Fresh fruit (focus on nonsweet, nonhybridized fruit and berries such as avocados, cucumber, zucchini, squash, lemons, limes, strawberries, blueberries, blackberries, mulberries, etc.)
- Nuts & seeds (in moderation and preferably soaked for easier digestion)
- Cold-pressed, unrefined oils (olive oil, hemp oil, flaxseed oil, coconut oil, ghee, etc.)
- Eggs from healthy, happy, grass-fed hens
- Wild-caught fish and meat from happy, healthy, pasture-raised and wild animals
- Raw, organic, cultured dairy (only if easily digested)

Eat Simple Food Combinations

—Food Combining for Easy Digestion—

If you experience bloating or any other discomfort after eating a meal, good food combining is an easy and effective way to increase the efficiency of the digestive process. Often, bloating and other digestive stresses stem from an inner imbalance of bacteria and yeasts. This imbalance can create all sorts of havoc when unwanted pathogens are being fed foods that feed them well instead of feeding you well in combinations that take much longer than they should to break down. If the digestive system is compromised or weak, putting foods that are not compatible together in the stomach supports fermentation, which creates an environment that feeds unwelcome organisms. As these organisms grow and reproduce, they create more waste—creating more work for the body.

The digestion of starches (potatoes, grains, and many root vegetables) requires alkaline conditions. The enzymes that digest protein thrive in acidic conditions. When we eat starches and proteins at the same time, we're asking our digestive system to be both alkaline and acidic—and neither the starch nor the protein gets broken down as efficiently if eaten without the other. By being mindful of a few favorable food combinations, we can reduce the likelihood of fermentation. As our body begins to work more effectively at breaking down foods, we have more energy that can be allocated toward other areas and needs. Eating foods that digest well together along with avoiding overeating, which leaves space in our stomach to do its job, can go a long way toward reestablishing and maintaining good digestion. There are many tips for efficient food combining, but to keep things simple, these are three essentials:

1. Eat fruits alone.
2. Eat protein with nonstarchy land and/or sea veggies.
3. Eat grains/starchy vegetables with land and/or sea veggies.

Avoid Overeating and Nighttime Eating

—Avoid Eating Until Full—

In our culture, it is very common to eat until full instead of eating until no longer hungry. When we eat until we feel full, we have already compromised our body's ability to digest our meal. Every time we eat, our stomach accomplishes three tasks:

1. It stores food and liquid by relaxing the stomach muscles to accept swallowed foods.
2. It produces digestive juices, which mix with the stored food and liquids.
3. It empties its contents into our small intestine.

The stomach needs space to do its job well, but if we eat until we are completely full, our overworked stomach is unable to properly mix the food it contains with its own digestive juices. This slows down the entire process, leading to food sitting, where it begins to ferment, creating sugars that feed microorganisms. Just as important, overeating leads to cell starvation by upsetting our metabolic balance—leading to the cycle of feeling undernourished, wanting to eat to deal with this feeling, and, as a result, supporting our body's increasing inability to pull and use nutrients from the food that is taken in.

If we are trying to heal our digestive system, refraining from eating too much is *crucial*—even if we are eating healthy, whole food. Easier said than done? It is truly difficult for many of us to eat small amounts. Our entire system is set up to consistently consume too much—from portion size (in both grocery stores and restaurants) to the almost exclusive focus on food and eating at family and holiday gatherings. Below are three tips to avoid overeating:

1. **Plan what you are going to eat *before* each meal.**
Though it varies slightly depending on the source (and likely varies slightly in each person, anyway), the stomach is about the size of two fists put together and can hold roughly under one quart of food/fluid. Make two fists, place them together, and imagine how much food you commonly take in during one meal. Typically, especially with our current portion sizes, the amount of food that we eat in one sitting is far more than we need. Planning what you're going to eat before sitting down at the table, keeping in mind the portion size in relation to your stomach size, greatly helps you to leave the table feeling satisfied instead of full—and allows your body to adequately break down and use the food that was consumed.

2. **Slow down.**
Although I just summarized in three very basic steps how our bodies deal with food, digestion is a complex process involving the cooperative concert of many hormones and enzymes. It takes about twenty minutes for our brains to signal that we've eaten enough, the amount of time most people take to eat a meal, so we are likely to overeat without even realizing it. Instead, we can focus on making meal time a pleasurable experience where we are calm, relaxed, and mindful of each bite. (Eating while stressed has a stamp of havoc all its own. It's always better to avoid eating while in "fight or flight" mode.) Digestion starts the minute food is placed into our mouths. Our saliva begins the breakdown process. Thorough chewing not only

slows us down, it allows us to more fully taste our food—making eating more enjoyable and helping us feel satisfied sooner.

3. Remember that you can eat again!

Try to move your mind away from the practice or standard of "eating everything on your plate" or "finishing everything on the table for a sunny day tomorrow" (two phrases that many of us grew up with). It is okay to stop eating when we feel satisfied! We can always eat again later.

—The 80/20 Goal—

The "80/20" goal is an easy guideline, spanning several different dietary traditions, that makes a variety of dietary practices more manageable.

- Aim to fill your plate with 80 percent land or sea veggies with the remaining being a heavier food.
- Eat until you are 80 percent full, leaving 20 percent of your stomach free to do a good job breaking down the food that you take in.
- Focus on health-supporting food choices 80 percent of the time so that you can fully enjoy any indulgences the remaining 20 percent.

—Daytime Eating—

I once read that the optic nerve is activated by sunlight and that its stimulation, in turn, stimulates digestion. I don't know this to be absolutely true, but after I research any subject enough, one of my favorite things to imagine is how tribal communities would have lived (by the mandates of nature) before modern tweaks.

Before man-made light, it seems unlikely that people in natural settings would have eaten past sunset. It wasn't until fairly recently in the 1600s that it became the norm to eat three meals a day, and, shortly after, a reshuffling of the meals—due to work/time constraints—made the evening meal (now called "dinner") the largest meal of the day. When it was customary for only one or two meals to be eaten, it was understood that going to bed while the body was still digesting any food at all was detrimental to both quantity and quality of sleep—and resulting health. Though I'll write more about the body's cleansing efforts and routine in Chapter 4 (p. 55), I'll briefly mention here that the body cannot give its full energy to vastly different processes at the same time. During the day, it is designed to be up and moving; to be taking in, breaking down, and using nutrients. During the night, the body is designed to cleanse and repair. If it has to continue dealing with nutrient intake, the processes of resting and renewing don't receive the full attention they deserve.

From the time of well-known Hippocrates and other health advocates of that period to more modern nutritional gurus, health-improving ideas and topics have been tossed around. These various health advocates, across hundreds of years, have observed and presented the same or similar information based on fundamental and uncompromising natural laws. Still, a look at the world around us reveals a present-day norm that greatly defies biological design. Understandably, it is difficult in many ways to adjust the mind and body to a different daily routine. However, adapting to a new (yet very old) lifestyle offers gains that are far-reaching (for ourselves, our loved ones, and our planet) and that, alone, hopefully makes change seem a bit more lovable.

Allow Your Intuition to Be Your Guide

—Releasing Dogmatic Approaches—

Everything, as in *everything*, is dynamic! All that is in, on, within, and about this world is always changing. Flowing with the changes— following those inner, intuitive nudges to do and/or try something different as it relates to what feels best for our life path—is . . . well, to put it very simply—good! Through working with others in the area of nutrition and health, I repeatedly discover that it is really easy for people to fall into the pattern of following different dietary protocols with "the strictness." Many people make a decision wrapped around an identity—"I'm a vegan, or a raw foodist, or I follow this plan or these guidelines"—as if their lives and sense of self depend upon it. When I first began this whole-food journey, I had the following general goals and visions at the fore: to gain more clarity, to feel more vibrant, and to help others (as well as our planet) do the same. Holding onto this vision throughout my learning process has allowed me to shift with ease when my body and my being suggest that changes are needed. I've also learned through the years that isolated and mass-produced nutrients are rarely a sound replacement for real food. There are ample amounts of supplements to make up for the nutrients that the primary staples of various dietary protocols lack. Yet, without walking too far into a vast (and sometimes emotionally loaded) arena, there are factors upon factors that have never been, are not, and will never be able to be bottled or put into pill form. There are countless considerations when extracting a component of something for which we can't even begin to imagine the process of creation. That said, because so much of our food is growing in depleted soil, there may be certain nutrients that we're not always getting enough of. If this is the case, consider whole foods–based supplements. For example, acerola cherry and camu berry powder are both rich in vitamin C; and herbal infusions (which I'll write more about later) are a great way to increase our mineral intake.

There is so much information to be tossed around when it comes to nutrition, but my goal with this book is to keep things short and simple, so I'll wrap up with this: It makes sense that we are designed to eat in the way our ancestors did—before the introduction of farming practices to our more modern ways of living. After studying and witnessing the implementation of countless dietary programs and paradigms throughout the years, very few have come close to so reliably affording the type of results that a whole-food, ancestral, biologically fitting diet offers. Every person is different! We are all on such unique and individual paths, with unique and individually tailored lessons. Blindly following another person's advice will likely never be as effective as incorporating into our lives what feels good and right—and then allowing *our* internal guidance system to lead us in making decisions that are best suited for our own well-being. Clear and strong intuition never guides in a shady way. Learn to recognize the energetic cues of your larger self—the "yeses" and the "noes"— and to trust in your ability to make changes for your greatest good and journey.

Nourish Intentionally with the Spirit of Love and Gratitude

Food is such an amazing and beautiful component of our earthly lives. Energetic transfer is a fluid, awe-instilling process that, as we become more centered, grounded, and aware, begins and continues to open up new and divine dimensions. We realize that food is not just food in its physical expression. It becomes the essence of what it was and what it will become, carrying with it—into our cells, into our sense of selves the energy that it has been imbued with throughout its journey. If food has been grown, harvested, and handled in the kitchen with a hurried, mindless, or unappreciated presence, it brings to us this energy. If food has been grown, harvested, and handled with the slow, engaging spirit of love and gratitude, it brings to us this energy.

The journey of food, from forest or field to plate to *being*, is full of wonder and magic. It grows, nourishes, and sustains us in ways that are both miraculous and often taken for granted. Becoming attentive and, as an inevitable result, grateful deepens our awareness of and appreciation for life and the responsibility that we each have to care for the world around us. Both then and now, the ritual of food has played an influential role in connecting us to Source and Spirit (however we wish to identify, name, or envision this). Whether through preparation, ceremony, blessing, intent, or symbolism, meal making is wordlessly recognized as an act of togetherness and devotion. When we softly step back from the rush of our daily goings-on and consider that the energy of our food may come from, and through, something far beyond and bigger than us, our awareness begins to shift. This shift will hopefully translate into us all becoming more mindful of how essential it is to actively care for and love our environment, families, and selves.

Following the five foundational nourishment general guidelines above—eating food in the state that nature creates and gives it to us while eating a wide variety of foods and tailoring other food items and/or processing methods to our specific bodily needs—will provide us with the array of nutrients we need to function optimally. Gradually—as we begin to pay attention to how we feel when we nosh on food that has spent time in a factory or years on a shelf, when we overeat, eat late at night, down a few funky combinations, or habitually eat while hurried or stressed—the above guidelines won't require much thought, and health will improve effortlessly. Regardless of which foods we choose to nourish our body with, the larger, more-encompassing journey is about creating change—for ourselves and for our planet—through making conscientious and respectful decisions in *all* of the ways that we choose to live our lives. Supporting good people with good practices who are providing good food helps in a big way to encourage this change.

Everyday Eating

Around here, there is a lot of playful banter about my aversion to measuring. I love looking through recipe books, but I have never followed a recipe. Exactness isn't something that I'm drawn to in the kitchen. Instead, I glance over recipes to get the general idea of the meal and then put together something that typically omits ingredients that I'm not resonating with or adds in more of the flavors that I enjoy. Meal preparation should be fun—and fun, to me, means having a lot of creative wiggle room. Honoring this sense of carefree magic in the kitchen and keeping with the theme of simplicity, I have created this section to present a small handful of easy, everyday ideas (none of which require measuring spoons or cups).

—Morning Ritual—

Whether it's a glassful of lemon juice in water, a mug of gut-soothing bone broth, or a simple cup of tea, it feels good to begin each day with some sort of nourishing ritual. I love starting the day with a balancing, earthy drink. I usually blend up a green smoothie, and, when I have planned for it the night before, I'll either drink a cup or two of herbal infusion or add some of this deep-steeped brew in with the smoothie ingredients. The days that I include a nutrient-rich infusion in the morning mix, I can feel enough of a difference that it deserves special attention.

Herbal Infusions

The green-drink bandwagon continues to gain members and momentum, and with good reason: these drinks offer nutrients that have become increasingly difficult to attain through our daily meals. Making a daily green juice or smoothie, however, can be time-consuming, and fresh produce isn't always available. Thankfully, there is another way to receive a sustaining array of vitamins and minerals   herbal infusions.

Regardless of how well we eat, our foods no longer contain the nutrients that they once did when grown on more fertile, nourished land. Most of our bodies are in need of extra vitamins and minerals, yet even naturally sourced nutrients in pill form can be difficult for our bodies to absorb and use. An herbal infusion, which is different from a tea due to the greater quantity of herbs used and longer steeping time, is a therapeutic brew that provides a large amount of bioavailable nutrients. A notable illustration of this difference is that a cup of nettle tea contains around five to ten milligrams of calcium, while a cup of nettle infusion contains between two hundred to five hundred milligrams of calcium, depending on the amount of herb used and infusion time. This significant increase in nutrients being pulled from the plant matter makes an infusion more medicinal. Because they are both cleansing and restorative, infusions are excellent allies to support functional wellness. They help to encourage balance. Like all other living beings, each plant has its own unique energetic imprint, which blends with our own to help support subtle shifts. It is common to begin to feel more connected with our natural world and to crave these rich, nourishing brews after drinking them for a few weeks. Below are two good plants to start with for making infusions.

Nettle

Strengthening the kidneys and adrenals, a quart of nettle infusion a day supports a significant increase in energy. With ample amounts of protein and an abundance of vitamins and minerals, this rich, earthy drink provides a strong foundation for overall vitality.

Red Raspberry

I was introduced to red raspberry leaf during my second pregnancy, when a lady at a farmers market thoughtfully handed me a bag. I quickly developed a connection with and appreciation for the bitter, nutrient-intense brew that it creates. Red raspberry leaf is often recommended to drink during the last trimester of pregnancy to help tone the uterus and support a strong milk supply. With its myriad of nutritional offerings, including a high concentration of vitamin C and a generous amount of bioavailable calcium and iron, the benefits from drinking red raspberry leaf infusion reach beyond the realm of birthing preparation—making it another reliable herb to help support foundational wellness. Creating an herbal infusion is quick and easy:

- Fill a glass quart jar with dried herbs. Add about an ounce by weight or a cup by volume.

- Pour hot water over the herbs and cover with a tight-fitting lid or a saucer to keep steam and volatile oils from escaping.
- Allow this infusion to sit for at least four hours to extract the vitamins and minerals.
- Strain and enjoy!

Infusions can be stored in the refrigerator for a couple of days.

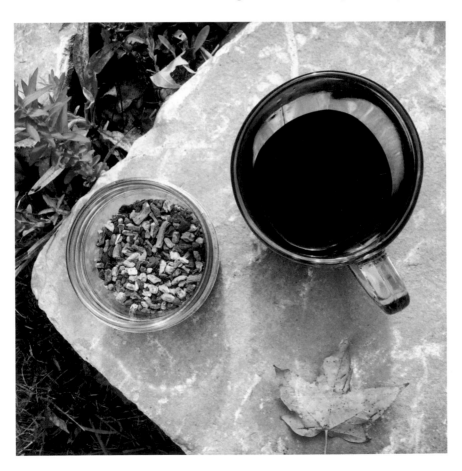

Four Easy Meal Ideas
Smoothies, Soups, Salads, Stir-Fries

No, I didn't plan on them all starting with the letter *s*, but it's convenient that they do. It makes them easy to remember. These four simple meals are nutrient-packed, easy to digest, quick to prepare, and can be tweaked for individual preference and variety. Again, these are not specific recipes. They are open-ended, foundational meal suggestions for those who are trying to eat less processed food but don't want to follow complex recipes or meal plans. At the beginning of each section, you'll find the general instructions for each meal, followed by ingredient combinations that you can put together in any amounts and ways that sound good.

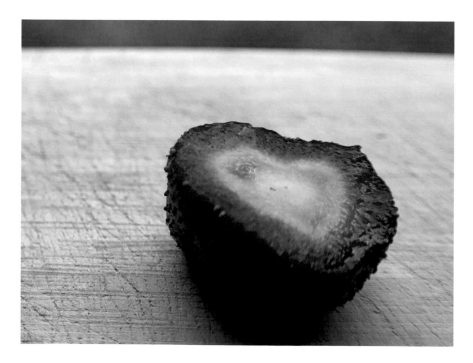

Smoothies

Or, more specifically, green smoothies. (I didn't want to mess with the quadruple *s* lineup!) It is really rare that I blend up a smoothie without tossing in a few handfuls of leafy greens. Greens are nutrient powerhouses, and blending them into a smoothie is an incredible and easy way to include them in our daily meals.

How to:

In a blender, combine any wild and/or leafy greens with fresh fruit and enough liquid to blend well. (A few ideas for blending liquid are water, coconut milk, almond milk, green tea, mint tea, green juice, or herbal infusion.)

Smoothie Combinations:

Plum-Berry Chard	Tropical Dandelion	Green Tea and Pear
• chard	• dandelion greens	• green leaf lettuce
• red or green leaf lettuce	• frozen mango	• fresh mint
• plums	• frozen pineapple	• cucumber
• berries (any)	• water, green juice, or coconut water	• pear
		• green tea
Orange Dream	**Simple Strawberry**	**Summer Love**
• mixed greens	• spinach	• spinach
• sorrel	• strawberries	• fresh mint
• orange	• almond or coconut milk	• cucumber
• lime		• watermelon
• coconut milk		• strawberries
		• avocado

Chocolate-Mint Mocha	Green Lemonade	Just Peachy
• Bibb or Boston lettuce • spinach • fresh mint • frozen banana • grass-fed ghee or coconut oil • cocoa powder • vanilla stevia • black coffee • coconut milk	• baby kale • lemons or limes • celery • apple • stevia, honey, or another natural sweetener	• any greens • frozen peach • coconut milk
Chocolate-Covered Cherry • any greens • frozen pitted cherries • frozen banana • carob or cocoa powder • almond milk	**Mojito** • Bibb or Boston lettuce • fresh mint • limes • stevia, honey, or another natural sweetener • rum extract (optional)	**Piña Colada** • spinach • frozen pineapple • rum extract (optional) • coconut milk

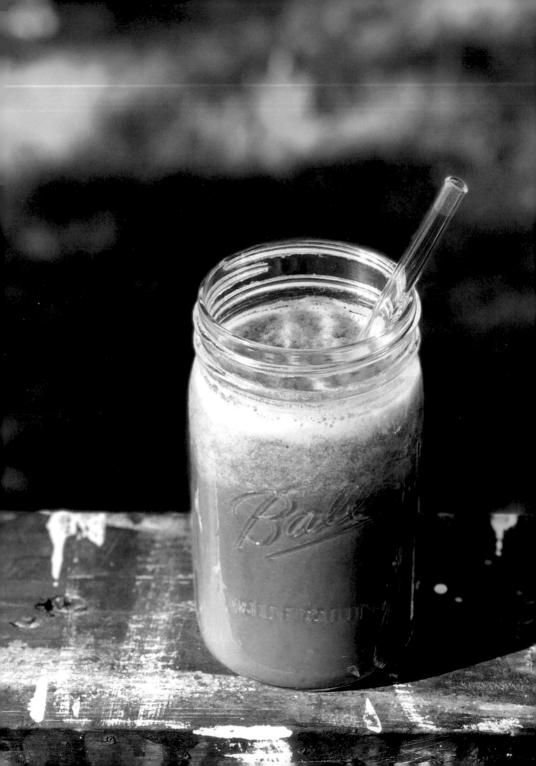

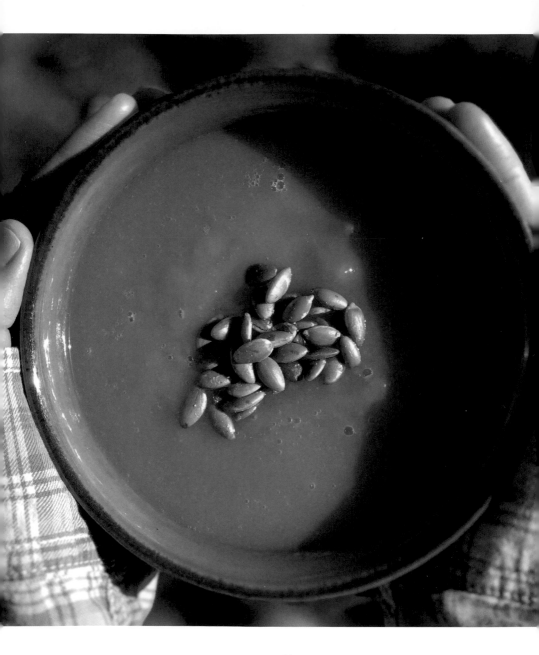

Soups

I get excited about soup! There are few meals as comforting or as nourishing. Part of what makes soup so balancing is that it's easy to digest, which simultaneously frees up the body to heal while providing nutrients. Occasionally, I'll make a soup with an array of whole ingredients in a broth base, but blended soups take the balancing act up a notch or two in my world, so soup ingredients often find their way to our kitchen's Vitamix. I'm most familiar with the below combinations as blended brews, but you can also make them in a broth base or even partially blended. Soups are vastly customizable. If you want a thicker soup, use less liquid and more veggies—or more liquid and less veggies for a thinner blend. Creamier? Add some coconut milk to the mix. For added nutrition, try a high-quality bone broth as the blending base. If your bowl is missing something, seasoning adds an entirely different and fun element to explore and enjoy.

How to:

Chop any combination of fresh land/sea veggies, leafy greens, and herbs. Cook (in just enough broth or water to cover) until tender. Season. Blend.

Soup Combinations:

Creamy Kale and Cauliflower	Sweet Beet	Wild Ramps and Celeriac
• cauliflower	• beets	• ramps
• kale	• sweet potato	• celeriac
• onion	• carrots	• parsnip
• lemon juice	• garlic	• leeks
• sea salt	• coconut cream	• sea salt
• black pepper	• sea salt	

Green Pea and Mint	**Cream of Cauliflower**	**Roasted Butternut Squash**
• green peas • onion • celery • mint leaves • sea salt	• cauliflower • onion • garlic • coconut cream • sea salt	• butternut squash (roasted) • carrots • onions • garlic • sea salt • black pepper • (cinnamon, ginger, and/or nutmeg)
Broccoli and Leek	**Wild Greens**	**Cauli-Cress**
• broccoli • leeks • onion • garlic • coconut cream • sea salt • black pepper	• dandelion greens • cauliflower • onion • garlic • sea salt	• cauliflower • watercress • leeks • garlic • sea salt
Carrot and Coriander	**Arti-Sunchoke**	**Summer Squash**
• carrots • fresh coriander • onion • coconut cream • fresh ginger • sea salt	• artichokes • sunchokes • leeks • garlic • fresh thyme • lemon juice • sea salt	• summer squash and/or zucchini • fresh basil • onion • garlic • lime juice • sea salt

Salads

It is difficult to go wrong with a mix of fresh, whole foods in one bowl. Salads are a symphony of colors, textures, and flavors—celebrating foods that are simple and straight from the earth. Many of us are used to salads being served before a main meal, but a salad *as* the main meal? Sure! A salad can be a blend of nearly any ingredient, in any amount—making it an easy dish to create as light or as hearty as wanted.

How to:

Combine any mix of leafy greens, veggies, fruits, proteins, nuts, or seeds. Add in a spoonful or two of fermented veggies, a drizzle of cold-pressed oil, lemon juice, or fresh herbs for increased nutrition and flavor.

Salad Combinations:

Spring Salad	Greek Salad	Butter Leaf and Fig Salad
• spring greens mix or green leaf lettuce • turkey bacon • red onion • steamed asparagus • strawberries • pecans	• romaine lettuce • cucumber • tomato • red onion • bell pepper • kalamata olives	• butter lettuce • roasted or steamed broccoli • red onion • fresh or dried figs • walnuts
Summer Salad	Classic Chef Salad	Smoked Salmon Salad
• cucumber • avocado • tomato • fresh peach	• romaine lettuce • baby spinach • hard-boiled egg • diced chicken • cucumber • shredded carrots • red onion	• spring greens mix • smoked salmon • green olives • cucumber • blueberries • dill

Fall Salad	Crunchy Waldorf Salad	Easy Taco Salad
• butter lettuce • roasted butternut squash • roasted carrots • apple slices • golden raisins • scallions • pumpkin seeds	• snow or sugar snap peas • celery • apples • red grapes • walnuts	• romaine lettuce • avocado • cherry tomatoes • onion • red bell pepper • seasoned grass-fed bison • plantain chips
Winter Salad	**Simple Green Salad**	**Broccoli and Mango Slaw**
• baby spinach • pasture-raised chicken • red cabbage • sweet potato • roasted or steamed cauliflower	• cucumber • celery • green peas • green pear • avocado • fresh basil • pistachios	• broccoli-carrot slaw mix • red bell peppers • fresh basil • mango • sliced almonds or cashews

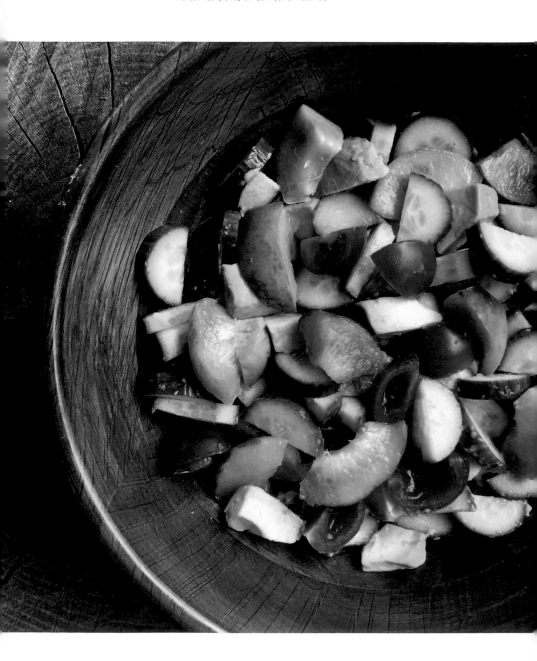

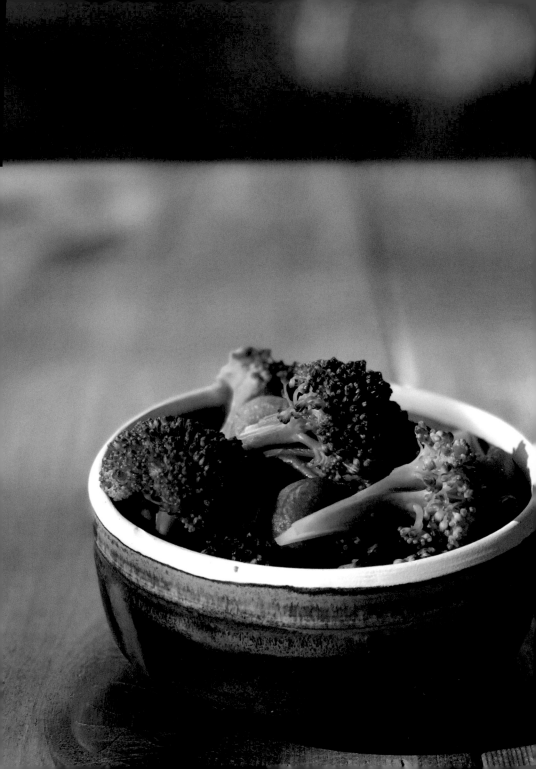

Stir-Fries

I am a huge fan of one-pan meals. Stir-fries or "steams," as we don't always use oil or high heat—sometimes just adding ingredients to a pan and letting them all steam together—are a staple meal around our home for two reasons: there are endless combinations of ingredients that taste well together, and they don't require a lot of time or attention. The combinations below list the main ingredients. You can further flavor any meal with a sauce or squeeze of citrus, top with or mix in pesto, drizzle with cold-pressed oil, stir in spices, or simply sprinkle with sea salt.

How to:

Stir any mix of chopped veggies and other ingredients in a pan over heat with a little bit of oil for high-heat cooking or just water for more of a steamed meal.

Stir-Fry Combinations:

Cashew Chicken	Bok Choy and Shiitake	Simple Broccoli
• pasture-raised chicken • scallions • celery • snow peas • cashews	• bok choy • carrots • scallions • shiitake mushrooms • sesame seeds	• broccoli • onion • cashews
Red Pepper and Kale	**Collard Greens and Apricot**	**Sweet Potato and Kale**
• kale • red pepper • onion • garlic	• collard greens • pasture-raised chicken • red pepper • dried apricot	• sweet potato • broccoli • kale • garlic

Cabbage and Apple	Green Bean and Bison	Summer Garden
• red or green cabbage • carrots • apple • onion	• green beans • carrots • bison, steak strips or ground • onion	• zucchini • yellow squash • sugar snap peas • carrots • onion
Turkey and Swiss Chard	Asparagus and Sunchoke	Spicy Spinach and Cauliflower
• pasture-raised or wild turkey • swiss chard • onion • garlic • currants • pine nuts	• asparagus • sunchokes • leeks • garlic	• cauliflower • spinach • onion • (sriracha or buffalo chicken sauce)

Keep in mind that the above are all just simple, quick, easily customizable ideas. I'm hoping that the larger takeaway is that meal prep doesn't need to be difficult or full of complex instructions or long lists of ingredients. It can be as easy as throwing whatever real, Earth-made foods that you have sitting on the counter or resting in the fridge into a blender or a pan. Feeling that meal making isn't such a chore goes a long way toward keeping us from loading our carts with a lot of prepared, packaged foods—and keeping meals fresh and whole.

-Creating Change-

- Go through the food in your home. Think about where it came from and how it was processed. Keep the foods that are Earth-made and whole and find a new home for everything else. Continue to keep these whole-food principles in mind while you shop, focusing on only bringing home foods that have not been processed.

- Pay attention to the types of foods that you eat together and try to focus on simple combinations. Also notice when you start to feel satisfied, instead of full, and save the rest for later.

- Set a time for your last meal of the day. Leave at least a couple of hours between this meal and the time that you go to bed so that your body can rest instead of digest.

- Create a special space while eating. Focus on nourishing your body and begin each meal with thoughts or words of gratitude.

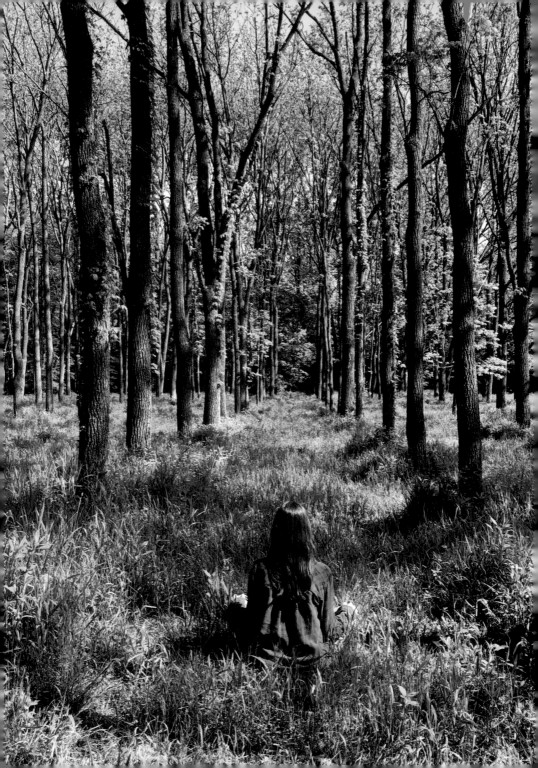

2

I Am Relaxed (Breath)

⋙⋙ ⋘⋘

"Please come home. Please come into your own body, your own vessel, your own earth. Please come home into each and every cell and fully into the space that surrounds you."

—Jane Hooper, poet

Breathing for Body and Mind

Without it, we would only live for a few minutes, so bringing up how important breathing is seems unnecessary—and yet some of us have forgotten what full and unguarded breathing feels like. As our lungs actively interact with the world around us, we experience the miracle and magic of being physically alive, but breathing in a way that makes us *feel* truly alive—that calls out to our tissues, our bones, our nerves, and every cell—frequently takes a back seat.

Breathing with a relaxed, open core and allowing the endless supply of energy that effortlessly arrives through this always-present process didn't require a lot of thought during childhood. We didn't have to plan for or practice our breathing; it just was. While this variety of deep, health-supporting breathing might occasionally be set to the side these days, it is never out of reach. With a little effort, it can be relearned and remembered.

Breathing is an involuntary function, yet distinct because it is a function over which we have voluntary control. It is difficult to control hormone release or digestive function, but we can inhale more deeply, retain our breaths for longer periods of time, and release more fully with a little conscientious effort. Our whole body breathes, and our whole body—every part of it—is affected by how we breathe. Our bodies want to breathe in the way that they are meant to—with a deep, fluent, easy rhythm, and with the steady goal of bringing oxygen to every cell, nourishing all parts and pathways. The natural health community commonly presents methods and supplements to better oxygenate our bodies, but instead of buying expensive products, why not relax into the all-around-us and ever-present source? Deeper, fuller (free!) breaths.

Many disorders are created or worsened through not having enough oxygen moving through the body. And, in turn, many can be cleared up through paying attention to our inhales and exhales. It sometimes seems as though the most basic ways to bring about balance are also some of the most neglected. Rethinking something so automatic and routine might seem a little elementary, yet it can be life-changing. Aside from the very essential, somatic role of bringing oxygen to our cells and releasing carbon dioxide, breathing plays a role in relaxing, strengthening, and healing our bodies.

Full and mindful breathing sends a "simma down now" (delighted to be working this SNL reference into the mix) message to our brain, which then travels to the rest of our body. Deep breathing lowers heart rates and decreases blood pressure. It calms and steadies the mind, leading to an inner sense of peace, awareness, and openness to what is around us. When our mind is tranquil, our perception and insight take on new depth, increasing creativity and our ability to work through issues. Breathing is an incredible way to help manage stress and stress-related conditions. Our lymphatic system, immune system, blood, organs, and physiological function are all strength-ened through breath. Deep breathing enhances circulation to the brain, heart, and liver. It can support or improve physical balance and alignment. It improves our digestion, nourishes our nervous system, and supports our lungs. When all parts of the body are oxygenated, toxins are released, tension and anxiety dissipate, uneasy feelings are cleared and transformed, and energy is improved. Amidst the foundational practice of breathing deeply, all of these things work together, with quickness and in so many ways, to bring about bal-ance and healing to both our bodies and our minds.

Breathing for Soul and Spirit

There are few things within our physical awareness that connect us to the nonphysical aspect of our being as completely as our breath. The process of moving air through and around our bodies somehow seems like more than an essential, biological function.

Breath *is* life. Spirit flows through our deep inhalation and release.

Various healing systems and teachers across different time periods and cultures have been aware of the healing benefits of breath—many believing that the breath is a link between the physical body and the ethereal mind, and that spiritual insight can be attained through conscious, controlled air exchange. As we slow down to observe our breathing, we cozy up to the experience of just being, right here, right now. This present moment is the moment that we are living in. Our breath grounds us in the company and potential of each of these current moments. Many of us intuitively know and understand how important it is for us to take time to still our minds, to be fully present, to connect with our bodies and our surroundings, and to breathe—deeply. We often become so wrapped up in personal expectations, achievements, and requirements that we neglect to focus on what is essential, what is with and near us in this very instant. Breathing can be a chance for us to come home to our own being and to the divine that is within us. It quiets the chaos and allows a core-emanating acceptance for *the perfection* of where we're at in our journey to surface.

Letting Go

Mindful breathing offers us the opportunity to inhale what fills us, what brings us peace and joy, and to exhale what no longer serves us. It aligns the body and the soul in quiet conversation. Through deep, complete, conscientious breaths, we can release the need for control, we can let go of our internal dialogue, we can free the expectations and evaluations that we have for and of ourselves, our lives, and of others. We can simply close the door, if only for a few minutes, and rest in the nourishing, sustaining tranquility of each moment that we are softly with. The process of breathing while releasing combined with envisioning and allowing offers up a quick and reliable path to get from wherever we are to wherever we want to be.

Being still isn't often an esteemed focus in our culture, yet it is often through this hushed space that spiritual guidance is most recognized and received. Through stillness, we are able to step away from our near-constant stream of thoughts and emotions and more deeply open up to our divine, instinctive selves and surroundings. We have a gift in our breath, and it is in graceful service within each of us every moment of every day. Our breath is a steady, gentle reminder that, when still enough to listen, is whispering, "now . . . now . . . and now." It speaks in clear and curative ways when we devote our time and attention to focusing on and being present with it. Each moment is ours to choose how we want to access and use our breathing to enhance our experience of living. Our deep, steady circulation of air—of life—connects us, expands us, heals us . . . and all it requires of us is that we settle down and settle in.

Remembering

After first waking up in the morning, have you ever noticed how you're breathing? Before the activities of the day take hold, I love lying in bed, noticing the full, calm, smooth way that my whole body is freely moving through and being cradled by each inhale and exhale. It feels like a remembering—an arrival to something familiar and wise. Whenever you naturally feel calm and relaxed—maybe during these early-morning moments, after a long bath, or while sitting outside on a warm, sunny day—take a moment to notice your breath. The pattern probably won't be controlled in any way. Your breaths won't be quick or curtailed. You'll likely notice deep, rhythmic inhales and exhales.

Breathing well isn't some new skill that we need to learn our way around. Breathing well is simply about moving our breath back down to the lower part of our body—where it started out and where it works best. Find a cozy spot, either sitting comfortably or lying down. Place one hand across your chest and one hand across your belly. Take a few deep breaths. Which hand moves? If the hand across your belly is moving first or mostly, then you're breathing from your core—the lower part of your body. If the hand across your chest is moving first or mostly, your goal is to work on moving your breath back down into your core. There are many reasons we might move away from belly breathing. Maybe we're sitting for hours every day in a position that has influenced the way we breathe over time. Maybe worry or fears have changed our breathing patterns. In a culture often focused on appearance, maybe some of us have purposefully shifted our breathing away from our stomach to the upper part of our body. Chest breathing is not as efficient as belly breathing. Belly breathing brings in more oxygen—which positively affects and influences all other areas and systems of our body. As the breath is consciously shifted back down below the chest, the muscles in the core strengthen and the body will remember this better-feeling way.

Three Simple Breathing Techniques

1. Creative Belly Breathing

This technique combines belly breathing with creative vision work to help bring balance to our body and being.

- Find a quiet, relaxed place to sit.
- Like above, place one hand on your chest and the other on your abdomen. As you breathe, notice how your upper

chest and abdomen are moving. Again, the hand on the abdomen should rise higher than the one on the chest

- Take a slow, deep breath in through your nose. You can imagine a cleansing and balancing energy flooding your body while thinking: *I am safe. I am balanced. I am whole. I am healthy. I am complete.*

- Slowly exhale through your nose or mouth (whichever feels the most natural and comfortable to you). As the air is released, imagine any negative energy leaving your body—any worries or stress evaporating into the air around you.

- Repeat.

2. Make Some Noise

At some point during high school, I started naturally doing this breathing technique (though I never thought much about it or referred to it as a technique at the time) that was so soothing that, all of these years later, it still occasionally drops in for an impromptu stress-relieving visit. I would breathe in, lifting my hands up and across the front of my face, as if gathering any unwanted energy. Once I reached the top, I would let my hands fall down the side, as if sweeping away this energy, while also breathing out, but not quietly. These exhales were loud—as if all the surrendered elements of that breath were throwing their hands up one last time while being escorted out. This may not be a technique that always feels comfortable while around others, but give it a try during a solo-style walk or a hot bath. As with all of these techniques, there's no right or wrong way to go about it. Just make some noise. There's something about a dramatic, audible release that feels as though it's working extra magic.

3. Breathing with the Trees

When I'm feeling the need to step away from people and buildings and constant movement and technology, I often find my way to the nearest wooded area. I sit or lie down on the ground, look up toward the swaying tops of the trees above, and begin to breathe. Deeply. I imagine the trees taking in my carbon dioxide and releasing oxygen; myself taking in oxygen and releasing carbon dioxide; and sometimes a piece of art that I once noticed and stared at for the longest while during a drive along the Blue Ridge Parkway. It was a photo of trees, and below it read, "We breathe for them. They breathe for us." So, I breathe for them, and they for me. It only takes a few breaths until we feel like one—rhythmically working together. This is one of my favorite practices. No time to step too far into the forest? No problem—just step outside your door. Find a cozy space anywhere on the ground . . . and breathe.

−Creating Change−

- Set aside ten to twenty minutes each day to practice one of these three breathing techniques. With whichever you choose, imagine restorative, loving energy filling you with each breath in, and anything that is holding you back leaving with each breath out.

- While creating still space for these breathing practices, try to focus on your immediate surroundings, allowing any concerns or mind chatter to drift away.

- Calm.com is a good online source for a variety of guided meditations and soothing background sounds.

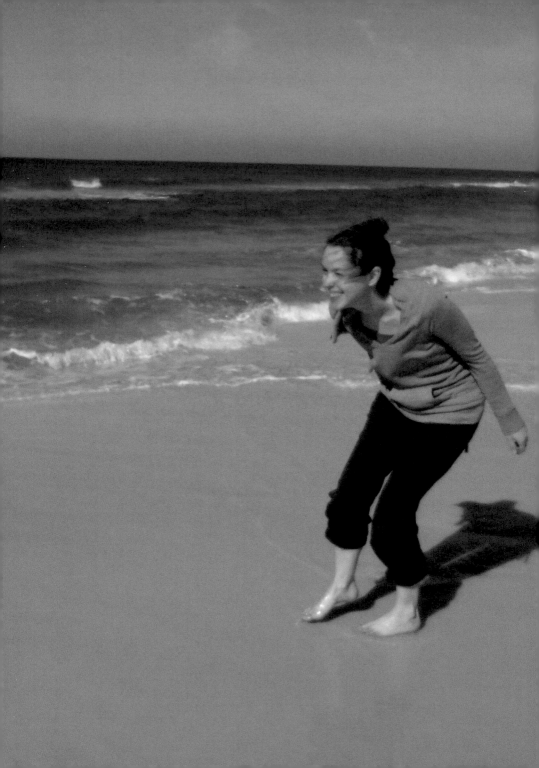

3

I Am Free (Movement)

≽≫⟩⟩ ⟨⟨⟨≼

"If you want to give birth to your true self, you are going to have to dig deep down into that body of yours and let your soul howl."

—Gabrielle Roth, dancer and musician

Flowing, stretching, reaching, releasing. Movement is freeing. It frees up the fluid in our lymphatic system. It frees up energetic tides. It frees up our mind from repetitive thought patterns. Of all of the essentials to health, exercise is probably the most talked about and focused on in our culture. Physical movement is vital to the well-being of our entire body and, when we're doing things that bring us joy, feels incredible. The feel-good capability of physical freedom aside, movement is a fantastic tool for managing and relieving a variety of chronic issues, more effectively dealing with stress, boosting the immune system, and improving the mind and mood. It increases the flow of oxygen, and helps to instill harmony throughout the body.

Lymph Flow

One of the lesser-mentioned ingredients to maintaining balance throughout the body is making sure that the lymphatic system is functioning well. The lymphatic system escorts toxins and excess fluid away from all bodily tissues. Our other circulatory system, which keeps blood flow moving, receives a lot of attention; yet the lymphatic system, with twice as many lymph vessels as blood vessels, is rarely brought up. These lymphatic pathways act as an internal vacuum. They connect up with every organ to absorb internal waste. If this flow is reduced, the fluid becomes thick and loaded with material trying to make its way out. The parts of the body that rely on it for elimination become weak and sluggish. Lymph flow is almost entirely dependent on movement, and, while any activity will help to eliminate fluid and waste, one in particular stands out when it comes to removing undesirable material—rebounding! Defying gravity, through jumping around, bathes our cells in fresh, clean fluid. A few minutes of jumping each day (even small, barely-there jumps) on a minitrampoline shakes those lymph nodes into waste-squeezing action. With each bounce, all the lymphatic valves open and close, and the change in gravitational force increases lymphatic flow. Alongside a nourishing, mineral-rich diet and deep breathing, rebounding is one of the best ways to cleanse our lymph of toxins, tone our digestive organs and muscles, and stimulate our endocrine system and brain.

Energy Flow

Throughout the past couple of decades, energy medicine has often been described as the next big thing in healthcare. There are so many tools and techniques to help shift and balance our energetic beings, and a variety of practitioners continue to crop up in both larger and smaller areas. Several US hospitals are now offering energy-focused therapies such as reiki to their patients—and many more provide patients with education about these types of healing techniques. Some might say that energy medicine is finally here . . . but it's really always been here. It's just returning to a place of deserved attention. Why? Because it's safe, effective, and easily accessible. All things are made up of energy. By connecting to the unseen, we work with and influence what we can see.

There are many different ways to support the smooth circulation of energy throughout and around our beings, and movement is one. Stillness can be amazing and really beneficial to our overall feeling of well-being. Too much stillness, however, can result in all of our systems taking on a slow, static presence. Physical movement supports good energetic flow. Likewise, good energetic flow supports our physical abilities. There are plenty of practices that focus on moving and balancing our life force energy, such as qi gong and yoga. Classes can be easily found for both in many areas, and books or video instruction can be found in any library or bookstore.

Our energy bodies have been evolving alongside everything else over millions of years, yet the world around us has rapidly morphed during a short period of time. We have energy systems that are acclimated to a wild world that few of us deeply interact with anymore. All day, every day, cell phone signals, Wi-Fi, and "smart" systems communicate with and influence biological systems that are designed to be communicating with the energetic symphony of a natural world. Our immune systems constantly deal with the unrecognizable, and, as a result, many are on constant alert. Daily stress pushes us into fight-or-flight mode in routine ways that cause us to regularly operate outside the realm of what would have been normal even a couple hundred years ago. The implications of these things are already unfolding and will probably continue to unfold in assorted ways as time moves forward, yet our bodies and beings continue on with such incredible intelligence. They are remarkably adaptable. They are constantly in conversation with the timeless wisdom of what is wild and what is still very much around and within us. Whether we are trying out a more hands-on technique, taking a break from the energetic influence of technology, or simply allowing the body to be in motion, recognizing the movement of energy as medicinal places the power over our health more securely in our own hands.

Mind Flow

"The fastest way to still the mind is to move the body."
—Gabrielle Roth, dancer and musician

After our house has quieted each eve, I like to head out for a walk. It is a practice that I have been enjoying for many years. While I appreciate all of the ways in which this evening stroll feels good, I appreciate it most for the ways that it influences and affects my mind. There are times when I spend the entire stretch of the night hike processing through the day's events—focusing on anything that seems to need further thought, thinking about goals, dreaming, and/

or simply feeling grateful. There are also times, especially when the terrain is rough, when I need to focus on the walk itself and my mind takes a couple of welcomed hours off from thinking about much else other than where my next step is going to be.

Wendy Suzuki, professor of Neural Science and Psychology at New York University and the author of *Healthy Brain, Happy Life,* says, "aerobic exercise can change the brain's anatomy, physiology—and function." Physical activity influences and affects our brains similarly to how it influences and affects our muscles. Through breaking down and then recovery, movement causes neurons to become stronger and more resilient. Physical activity has a positive impact on several components of mental presence and function, including things like memory, alertness, concentration, and creativity. Exercise also releases endorphins in our bodies, which dampen our perception of pain and trigger a positive feeling—making it a great and natural therapy for depression.

Moving Naturally

Older generations didn't have structured exercise routines as people in our current culture often do, because their lives naturally required an abundance of physical activity. Trips to the store or to a friend's house required a walk, smaller homes that made use of vertical space required several trips up and down stairs, sitting on the floor to eat called upon the dedicated use of leg muscles—often several times during a meal. There was no button to push for dishwashing, car washing, or lawn care. Food and water collection mandated much more than driving down the road to gather packages from grocery store shelves. The lack of modern-day conveniences supported strength in the bodies of these people, which is why functional movement-focused fitness programs are cropping up all over the fitness world today. There are many modern conveniences that we can trade in for opportunities each day to work and use our entire body. We can choose to walk or bike instead of drive to local spots around our community. We can set aside the leaf- or snow blower and pick up a rake or shovel. Cleaning our homes, planting a garden, mowing our grass, and walking the dog are all great physical activities. Using stairs instead of the elevator can offer up small cardiovascular workouts throughout the day. If you sit at a computer for much of your day, see if you can arrange your desk so that you have the option to stand up. Park a few blocks away from where you're going. Save money by avoiding expensive appliances designed to make life easier to instead make life simpler and more active. Add in a few fun, not-for-the-home activities such as swimming, hiking, paddle boarding, or rowing. These are just a handful of ideas, but there are countless ways to move naturally throughout the day. Whatever feels good and keeps your body moving—do that.

Letting Go and Letting In

"We have come to be danced
not the pretty dance
not the pretty pretty, pick me, pick me dance
but the claw our way back into the belly of the sacred, sensual
animal dance
the unhinged, unplugged, cat is out of its box dance
the holding the precious moment in the palms of our hands
and feet dance."
—*Jewel Mathieson, poet*

I do love the evening stroll that I mentioned earlier, but when I feel the need for a quickly balancing, midday break from the everyday routine, I often turn to dance. This form of meditation-through-movement is special enough to have a section all its own—and not just because I spend an impressive amount of time aimlessly flailing around the living room to a nostalgic mix of eighties tunes. My nephew who is nearing two years old has some moves, and when the music starts playing, he doesn't hold back. He reminds me that dancing—just like smiling or laughing—is something that emanates from our unguarded core.

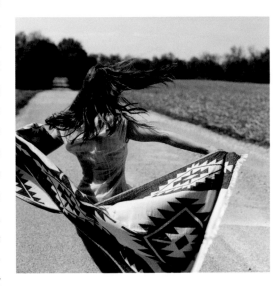

We don't have to think or plan it out. A good rhythm begins, and our bodies know what to do. They know how to push our thoughts to the side, to unveil, to unfurl. They know how to move energy around, how to balance . . . how to heal. Dancing strengthens bones and improves cardiovascular health. It is an accessibly great physical activity, but its goodness also has far-reaching effects for our minds. It releases tension and allows blocked energy to shift and flow more freely.

It seems clear that dancing is good for our bodies and our minds, yet there's something deeper and more inexplicable about it. Dancing harnesses the capability of movement, music, and intent to create experiences that inspire, engage, awaken, and activate. Connecting us with something central and sacred, to the flow and rhythm of life, dance reveals a portal for us to experience our own spiritual and physical fluidity in this universal journey of embodiment. It unlocks wisdom from deep within our bodies and offers us a different understanding of wholeness. Words can get in the way of good communication. Walking through a forest, lying against our Earth, embracing our partner, laughing, singing, star gazing—these all, as well, involve stepping outside of relating through words and ask that we attune to a rhythm that somehow unites us with all that is. Dancing is an invitation to fuel the power and joy in our connection to the always-in-motion universe. Through unrestrained movement, in the presence of an enlivening pattern and pulse, we can discover a home for expression, integration, and healing. Regardless of where you are or what your physical capabilities are in this moment, if any of this speaks to you, I encourage you to turn your favorite music on, turn the volume up, tune in to each part of your body, allow its story to unravel, to stretch out. Shake and shimmy any stagnant thoughts, unresolved feelings, or limiting beliefs to the surface. Wiggle and writhe them out and away. Keep your mind open and clear, listening only to the music and to the parts of your being that are communicating through movement. Acknowledge and release their mumbles and moans. Move fluidly toward the variety of passionate, inspired state of being that leaves you with little to focus on outside of the marrow of your unrestrained attendance and the remedial beat. You might find that some of the most connected moments and spirited ideas will find their way to you in this sacred space of letting go and letting in.

Balance

Physical activity is only one of several components to wholeness. It is only one element, in this physical realm, that affects our health. Our bodies require movement to maintain health, yet movement alone won't necessarily create lasting wellness. Even if we maintain a regular "workout" routine, exercise is not likely to magically tip the scale in favor of vibrancy and balance if our body is consistently dealing with materials that it doesn't know how to process (from food products, air, water, inadequate sleep, negative thoughts, and/ or sticky emotional baggage). True balance involves focusing on all areas of our life rather than focusing on getting to a place of well-being through fitness alone.

-Creating Change-

- To keep your lymph system pumping, make time to jump around each day. If you don't have a rebounder to jump on, walking is another effective way to increase lymph flow.

- Whether it's walking to the store, biking to work, raking the lawn, or handwashing dishes, try to work natural movement into your daily life as often as you can.

- Take an afternoon dance break (or several throughout the day). Start off by choosing just one or two of your favorite dance tunes and work your way up to a few songs each dance session.

4

I Am Renewed
(Rest)

"A good laugh and a long sleep are the best cures in the doctor's book."

—Irish proverb

Even if we're diligent enough to avoid intentionally sacrificing sleep for "catching up" or entertainment purposes, life has, at times, a humorous way of playing with our most well-intentioned aspirations. Flights leave early. Babies seem eager for the day to start. Projects, bills, chores, and deadlines keep us up later than anticipated. Some of us might deliberately stay up to bask in what may be the only handful of solitary minutes that we come across each day. These few treasured moments—while the children are asleep, the world is hushed, and the bliss of reconnecting with our own thoughts, if only for a short while—seem too important to lose to dreamtime hours. The next morning, however, finds us gripping

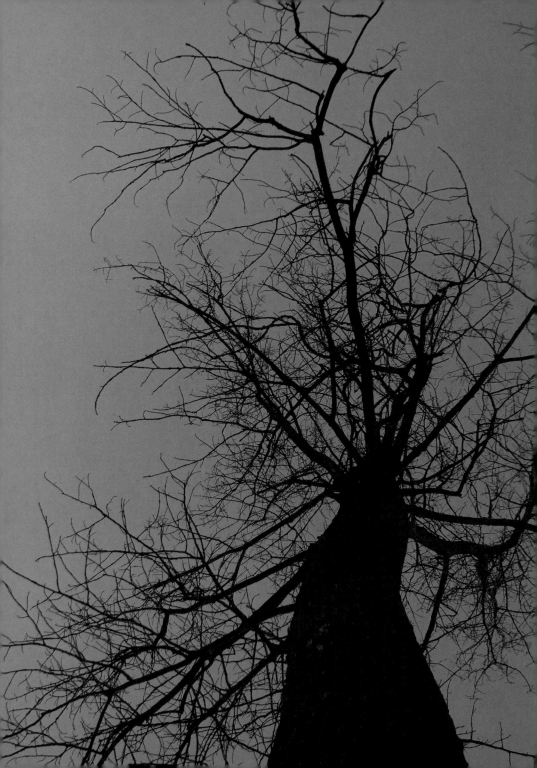

our pillow. No matter how much we enjoyed or appreciated the previous night's activities, we now regret this late-night extension. The bed becomes the most wonderful and inviting place in the world. We reach for the snooze button—another extension—and the cycle continues.

Why Sleep?

Historically, sleep was thought to be a passive state. Thankfully, new information is always unraveling and revealing itself, and sleep is now understood as a far-reaching activity for both our brains and our bodies, during which we dreamily dive into all sorts of growth and repair processes. It is a dynamic biochemical orchestration that is essential for the normal functioning of all of our biological systems. Sleep increases memory, boosts problem-solving skills, and, in general, helps us feel physically good with a calmer, more positive outlook facing the day ahead.

When sleep is consistently placed on the back burner, every bodily system is affected, in some way, trying to catch up and balance out. Physically, it becomes more of a challenge for the body to deal with moderate, daily stress. Immune function is compromised, impairing the body's ability to fight infection. Even a single night of sleeplessness can increase inflammation throughout the body. Mentally, all varieties of both short- and long-term memory are sacrificed or impacted. And it is no surprise that lack of sleep has emotional effects—intensifying depressive and/or psychological conditions that are already present and, in general, throwing basic emotional regulatory abilities to the wind.

Natural Rhythms

In our modern world, sleep can be thrown off course by the flip of a switch (literally). Before the invasion of modern-day appliances and conveniences, there were no alarms, clocks, televisions, radios, lights, smartphones, or other intense, biologically defiant technological gadgetry to put our circadian rhythms (physical, mental, and behavioral changes that follow a daily cycle) to the test. How might our nights be different if we spent ten to twelve hours with only star- or moonlight? Our bodies are designed to flow in synchronicity with the cycles of nature. Nature acts and moves according to rhythmic cycles influenced by the rotation of the Earth, sun, and moon. The sun rises, the sun descends, seasons spiral in and out, the moon waxes and wanes, and the ocean tides rise and fall. The activity and sleep cycles of all creatures around the globe—both plants and animals—are naturally influenced by these rhythms. Humans are designed, as well, to be rolling along to the beat of this mother drum—yet most of us have managed to step away, swayed by a different rhythm.

One of the most powerful external influences on our circadian rhythms is exposure to light and dark. The brain keeps track of light, as it shifts over the stretch of a twenty-four-hour period, through cells in the back of the eye. These cells send information about the length and brightness of this light to our "master clock," which is located in the brain and is responsible for coordinating all other biological clocks and keeping the body on a twenty-four-hour schedule. The master clock has several duties, one of which is to signal the production of melatonin, a sleep-supporting hormone with powerful antioxidant properties. Melatonin production begins about two hours before we begin to feel sleepy and continues throughout the night until shortly before we wake up in the morning. It acts as a messenger between the master clock and other circadian clocks in the body—each with its own rhythm that is coordinated by the master clock and largely determined by the twenty-four-hour cycle of light and dark. If our exposure to light and dark becomes irregular, these internal rhythms fall out of sync.

The light bulb is a neat invention—one that most of us use every single day and are grateful for—but sometimes I wonder if it hasn't been as influential in the story making of our collective health as processed food. Prior to the widespread use of electricity, people would go to bed shortly after sunset. The best hours of sleep for our bodies are between ten at night and six in the morning. During these hours, with the natural cycle of our internal clocks calling the shots, the body is designed to cleanse and repair. We might not feel the effects of occasionally staying up late, but consistently stepping away from this natural cycle is a recipe for shifts that could lead to more chaotic conditions.

Things to Consider for a Good Night's Rest (and Supporting Our Internal Rhythms)

Darkness

Sleeping in complete darkness (the variety of "pitch-black" that makes it difficult to see our hand in front of our face) is important for good production of melatonin. Even the most unassuming bit of light can interfere with our internal clock and disrupt the pineal gland's production of this hormone. Be mindful of keeping the lights off—even for brief periods throughout the night, such as using the bathroom. If you get up throughout the night, consider using a low, nonblue light, such as a Himalayan salt lamp, instead of a fuller-spectrum, brighter light. If you have street or neighbors' lights coming through your bedroom window that regular curtains aren't blocking, consider investing in some blackout drapes.

Sunlight

Exposure to natural, bright sunlight during daytime hours increases the production of melatonin and, in turn, helps to regulate our internal clock—promoting sound sleep cycles. If most of the day is spent indoors, try stepping outside more often—even if it's only for a lunch break or taking a roundabout way to the car after work. Not only does sunlight affect our internal rhythms, it helps our bodies create vitamin D, which helps to balance calcium in the blood and supports our immune system and healthy cell growth. Studies indicate that the majority of us would benefit from more of this vitamin and that enjoying the sun directly on our skin for just ten to twenty minutes a few times a week is enough to raise vitamin D levels.

Movement

Making sure that we are moving our bodies enough throughout the day (not around bedtime) will help to reinforce our natural "daytime-action and nighttime-rest" cycle. Find ways to exercise that are fun, that feel good, and that fit into your daily life in a way that they routinely happen . . . just don't lace up your dancing shoes too close to bedtime.

Eating

As mentioned in the Chapter 1 (p. 1), an empty stomach allows the body to shift into repair mode while it rests. If the body is busy breaking down food, it has less energy to direct toward nighttime functions and goings-on. To help support good-quality sleep, try to eat your last meal or snack of the day a few hours before bedtime.

Sound

Being unable to fall asleep because our neighbor's dog is barking or our partner is loudly snoring has an obvious impact on sleep quality. Our brains continue to register and process sound after we've fallen asleep, so even if noise doesn't fully wake us or seem to consciously bother us while not awake, it can still affect our quality of sleep. Creating a quiet space (or a space with soothing, natural sounds like the movement of water or leaves in the wind) can improve the amount and type of rest that our bodies receive each night.

Temperature

Light gets a lot of attention when it comes to circadian rhythms, but temperature plays a role, too. After stepping out of a sauna or a hot bath/shower, or after sipping a hot cup of tea, the small drop in body temperature, signals that it's time for bed.

Sacred Space

Our living space can greatly influence our minds. Simple, clutter-free spaces often have a calming effect. Keeping all sorts of unfinished projects and materials used for a variety of activities can keep our minds on the move and unable to easily slow down for a good rest. Eating and watching television are activities that sometimes find their way into the bedroom, but they can create a different feel for and energy around this area as well as bring in strong electromagnetic fields, which may influence our sleep quality. Using our bedroom solely for sleeping is one way that we can help to convince and assure our subconscious that this space is reserved for deep restoration.

Routine

Keeping a consistent day-to-day schedule helps to keep our biological clock regular and our sleep deep and restful. Regardless of whether we're able to stick to a routine, climbing into bed on the early side is worth the commitment.

-Creating Change-

- Make an effort to be in bed by 10 o'clock each night to support your body's natural cleanse-and-repair cycle.

- Each night, about two hours before bed, turn off bright lights from television, computer, and phone screens and turn down bright lights from bulbs. If you need to be on your phone, tablet, or computer screen during these hours, consider downloading a free app, such as f.lux, that is designed to adjust a display's color temperature according to location and time of day.

- Read through this chapter's list of things to consider for a good night's rest and address each one with your unique sleeping space in mind.

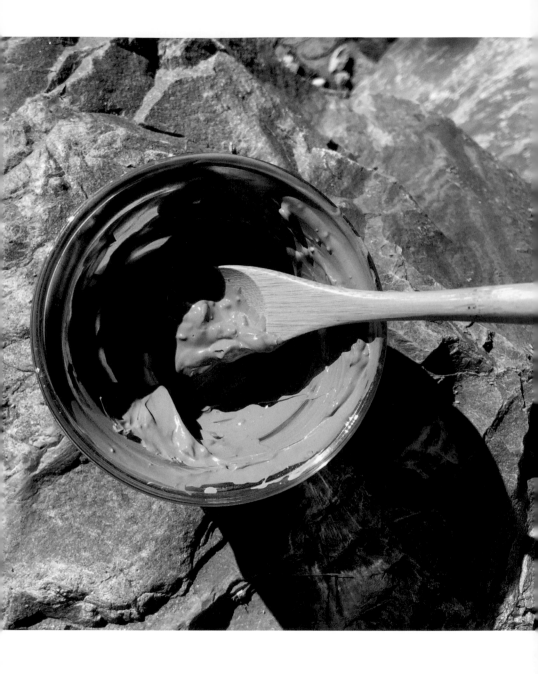

5

I Am Pure
(Cleansing)

※※〜〜

"There is more wisdom in your body than in your deepest philosophy."

—Fredrich Nietzsche, philosopher

All living things on our planet are continuously cycling through processes of cleansing. We live in an environment that is constantly throwing a lot of unnatural things our way, and there are practical ways to gently support our body's natural balancing efforts. The cleansing process is fairly straightforward; when the organs that are responsible for ushering out unwanted substances become overwhelmed, these substances find a place to hang out in our body—sometimes where weakness is already established. In an attempt to maintain optimal balance, the body orchestrates a purge—forcing out the things that do not serve it well—that shows up as some sort of turmoil, such as a fever, a cold, or feeling tired.

Eliminating through various channels is an ongoing, largely unnoticed process, yet most of us experience, from time to time, symptoms of a more acute and/or thorough removal. Fever reducers and cough suppressants are staples in many household cabinets and are routinely dispensed at the first signs of cleanup. While uncomfortable, these cleansing responses are quickly appreciated when they're understood as a healthy body trying to stay healthy. When these attempts to release undesired materials are repeatedly shut down through taking medicines to stop the process and ease the symptoms, materials that would otherwise be on their way out, with no place to go, might be driven deeper into the body.

When our body begins to let go of materials being held within it, it might look and feel like a disturbance to our entire being. This upheaval can even have a significant impact on our mind and emotions. It's sort of similar to cleaning our home spaces. When we begin to deeply clean a room, there is often a period when things look much worse than they did before starting the process. Things get moved around, dust fills the air as it is removed from resting spots, yet when this process is finished, the room looks and feels much better than it did before. Instead of approaching cleansing as a short, few-weeks stretch once or twice a year, during which a few herbs are taken or food intake is slightly tweaked, it's helpful to make clean living a daily way of life. Being mindful of decreasing the number of harmful things that we allow into our bodies is as important as being mindful of helping our bodies to eliminate what is already present— and what we cannot control allowing in.

It is difficult to fully heal without allowing our body to cleanse— and, at times, it is discouraging to feel as though our efforts to support our body and this process aren't producing quick or noticeable results. Knowing that we each have an unavoidable load of unwanted input from our environment, I have been open, through the years, to receiving information regarding effective support for the cleansing efforts of our bodies. I have never asked for the ideas or practices to be easy. The use of clay, both internally and externally, and releasing through sweat are both—easy *and* effective. These two strategies are inexpensive, and they don't require tracking down a lot of products or following complicated, time-consuming programs.

Clay

I am in awe of clay. Oftentimes, the most impressive finds are discovered through simple things and simple ways.

Eating Clay

Some people may underrate or entirely write off edible clay due to its simplicity, yet it is truly a beneficial gift from our Earth. Eating clay has been and is a common practice in many indigenous, nonindustrialized cultures. In his well-known book *Nutrition and Physical Degeneration*, Dr. Weston Price writes about the native cultures that he studied and their practice of routinely consuming clays and also of carrying clay with them to negate effects from any poisons they might come in contact with while traveling. Clay's negative electromagnetic charge gives it the ability to draw in and usher out positively charged toxins from the body, making it a powerful internal cleanser. It simultaneously gifts us an abundance of minerals in bioavailable form that very few of us are able to receive through our food, which is often grown in nutrient-depleted soils. Finding good-quality clay is important. Different clays have different qualities, and not all clays are mined with attention to purity. Research the companies that you source clay from well—not only taking note of the products that they offer, but also off-site reviews. How much and how often to eat clay will vary from person to person and should be guided through both research and intuition. Get to know the clay that you decide to use and decide what feels effective and right for you and your body.

Bathing in Clay

Clay's toxin-attracting capabilities aren't only useful *inside* the body. It can be used, just as effectively, to draw out unwanted elements from the outside. Again, because clay has a uniquely strong negative ion charge, it attracts things with a positively charged ion (most impurities are positively charged), like a magnet. To take a clay bath, simply mix 1 to 2 cups of clean, natural clay with warm water and enjoy a relaxing soak.

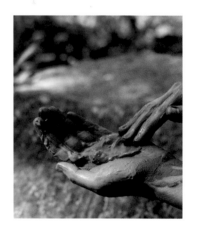

Sweating

"To sweat is to pray, to make an offering of your innermost self. Sweat is holy water, prayer beads, pearls of liquid that release your past. Sweat is an ancient and universal form of self-healing, whether done in the gym, the sauna, or the sweat lodge . . ."

—*Gabrielle Roth, dancer and musician*

Many people in our culture seem afraid to sweat. We go to great lengths to avoid the feeling of sweat-drenched clothing and bodies—even conditioning our inside air to avoid the natural detoxification that happens through sweating during the warmer months. The value and role of sweating, however, goes beyond temperature regulation. Our sweat escorts so much out of and away from our bodies. It's like taking a shower from the inside out. Both water-soluble and fat-soluble toxins are excreted through our sweat, so, unlike the release of mostly water-soluble toxins through our urine, sweat allows us to excrete things like heavy metals and radioisotopes, which are stored in our fat. The following is a quote from a study published in the *Archives of Environmental and Contamination Toxicology* in 2011:

> Toxic elements were found to differing degrees in each of blood, urine, and sweat. Serum levels for most metals and metalloids were comparable with those found in other studies in the scientific literature. Many toxic elements appeared to be preferentially excreted through sweat. Presumably stored in tissues, some toxic elements readily identified in the perspiration of some participants were not found in their serum. Induced sweating appears to be a potential method for elimination of many toxic elements from the human body.

Researchers from this study also noted that blood and/or urine testing might not accurately gauge the total body load of the material being tested for and that analyzing sweat should be considered as a further method for monitoring the accumulation of toxic elements. A couple of additional studies have found that endocrine-disrupting petrochemicals (like BPA) can be eliminated through sweat—and if you go looking for research linking sweating to detoxification, you'll probably come across a sauna detoxification project involving 9/11 rescue workers. From September 2002 through September 2005, more than five hundred of these rescue workers, the majority of them firefighters between the ages of thirty-five and forty-five, completed a sauna detoxification program. Below are the results:

> Before treatment, which averaged 33 days, they missed a median of 2.1 days of work per month and had 4.4 days of limited activity. Symptom severity scores—which rated 10 systems, including skin, respiratory, emotional, cognitive, and musculoskeletal—were high, and half of the participants were taking drugs to manage their symptoms. After this detoxification program, the number of days of missed work or limited activity fell to 0.2. Symptom scores dropped dramatically, and 84 percent of participants had discontinued all their drugs because their symptoms had cleared up. They also had significant improvements in thyroid function, balance, reaction time and even IQ!

Information from the New York Rescue Workers Detoxification Project and relating to Dahlgren, J., et al., "Persistent organic pollutants in 9/11 world trade center rescue workers: Reductions following detoxification," *UCLA School of Medicine, Occupational Medicine* indicates that there's something special about the regular use of saunas when it comes to releasing unwanted chemicals through our skin. In some cultures, saunas are taken as often as showers. An infrared sauna is especially beneficial, as it heats tissues several inches deep, possibly increasing its ability to help the body release stored materials. If having a sauna in your home is not an option, consider a membership at a gym with saunas. No access to a sauna? Find another way to sweat it out. They might not all produce the same type of dripping-with-sweat experience, but any type of activity—hiking, running, dancing, working outdoors—that supports an "outpath" through your skin will be beneficial.

A Special Gift for Women

Our menstrual cycle offers us a unique opportunity to cleanse. As our body begins its monthly process of shedding the lining of the uterus, it also integrates a whole-body release. The way that the moon cycle is reflected in our own moon-time cycles is stunning. The lunar cycle consists of twenty-nine and a half days—shifting from the waxing moon of increasing light to the full moon of complete illumination to the waning moon of decreasing light and beginning the cycle, again, with the waxing new moon of increasing light. It does not seem coincidental that the average length of a woman's cycle is twenty-nine and a half days, as well—and parallel to the moon's cycle, a woman's cycle shifts from new growth to the ovulation of full power and efflorescence into the energy of dissolution, and full-circle back into renewal.

In many tribes, women would separate themselves from the group during menstruation. They cycled together in a "moon lodge" while the men and grandparents temporarily took over caring for the children and other responsibilities. During this time, women were considered even more powerful and would focus their individual and collective energy upon meditation, transformation, reflection, decision making—and, in general, deeper truth. For many, this time also serves as an energetic source of strengthening the bond between our collective divine feminine energy.

It's not uncommon to hear women complaining about the inconvenience(s) of their cycles. However, if we shift our understanding of what menstruation is, what it symbolizes, and the ways in which it connects us to others and the world around us, we can better understand and lean into this time for the gifts of growth and change that come through release, reflection, and renewal. To honor this beautiful monthly offering, we can take time to support our bodies through eating warming and nourishing foods, spending time with nurturing friends, resting, quieting our mind (and our living space), and feeling grateful for the opportunity to surrender and channel so much through this special process.

–Creating Change–

- Decrease the amount of unwanted substances surrounding you through becoming more mindful about the materials and products you have or use in and around your home, including what you're applying to your skin and what you're consuming.

- Invest in a high-quality clay to help remove unwanted materials from your body.

- To help support the cleansing process, find a routine way to "sweat it out."

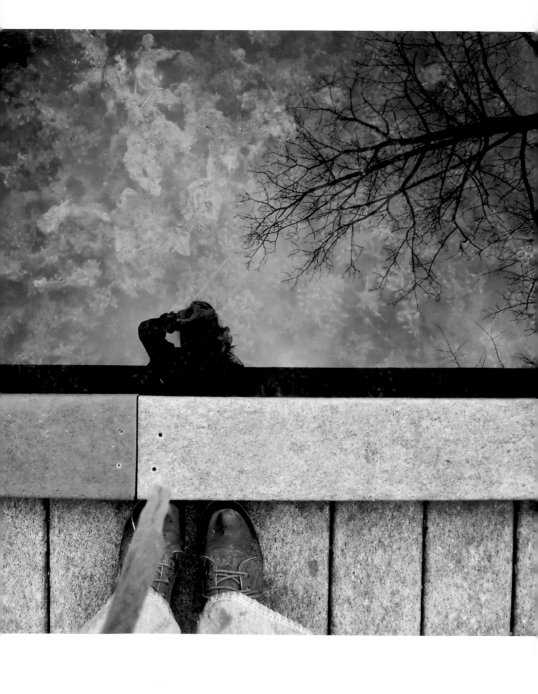

6

I Am Creative (Thought)

"From the moment I fell down that rabbit hole, I've been told what I must do and who I must be. I've been shrunk, stretched, scratched, and stuffed into a teapot. I've been accused of being Alice and of not being Alice, but this is my dream. I'll decide where it goes from here."

—Alice, in *Alice in Wonderland*

Thoughts and feelings are powerful gateways to change. The body is a dynamic construction that readily responds to the patterns of feeling and thought that are within and around it. Unhealthy attention can eventually express itself physically. Likewise, strong, happy, joyful attention helps to create and support a strong, happy, joyful experience. I liken the comparison of our minds to a garden. In a garden, caring for and focusing on the types of plants that we want in the space and constantly weeding out undesirable plants will support a healthy habitation. Similarly, through the consistent trimming back of fear-based, untrue and/or detrimental thoughts and focusing on the things which bring us joy and allow for and support truth, we each are cultivating a certain space for and presence of our soul—we each are the master gardener of our life.

With all of its colorful, ever-changing goings-on aside, when we reach further into the framework of life, energetic involvement becomes clearer and more substantial. One of the more compelling "intangible tangibles" involves the power of our own belief. What we *believe* to be true for our lives shapes our expectations. What we expect influences our experience. Our past thoughts have played a role in creating our present life. Our present thoughts will play a role in creating our future. Our subconscious mind accepts the things that we focus on most often—the things that we choose to believe. If we habitually choose to believe that our life is a certain way, then this is what we will identify with in the world. This is the situation, the reality that we, over time, will expect and most readily perceive. However, if we are willing to release that pattern and get cozy with, expect, and trust in a better-feeling, better-fitting idea, then this becomes the experience that we're more likely to recognize and resonate with. The present moment is always the most powerful. It is the only moment that we truly have. The past is over; it is behind us. We cannot change the past. It is ineffectual to punish ourselves in the present for things that occurred during a moment that will never exist again. The future has not yet arrived; it will always be in the process of arriving. *This* is the powerful moment that we have to create through our patterns of attention and beliefs—this one *right here*.

Forgiveness

Guilt, fear, resentment, regret—we all, at some point, get to deal with and process some (or all) of these weighty feelings in life. Regardless of what the issue is, many of our experiences are outer expressions of internal dealings and dialogue, but these dealings and dialogue can be refocused and released. For many, to move forward in any healing process, it is helpful to let go of the past, appreciate it for the lessons that it gifted, and forgive everyone, including yourself. You may not feel ready to forgive certain people or certain situations, but if forgiveness is something that is tugging at your soul as a way to help you move forward and beyond, the following is a good place to start. **Ho'oponopono** is an ancient Hawaiian practice of reconciliation and forgiveness. It is a very simple yet potent meditative path to releasing the energetic aftermath from past events.

Ho'oponopono *(ho-o-pono-pono)*

- I'm sorry.
- Please forgive me.
- Thank you.
- I love you.

(I like to add in "I forgive you" along with "Please forgive me.")

Through "I'm sorry," we're acknowledging whatever weights we are feeling in our life while also acknowledging our responsibility in relation to them. Through "please forgive me," we're asking for forgiveness and compassionate energy to surround these weighty-feeling experiences or events and any questionable role we've had in them, known or unknown.

"Thank you" expresses gratitude for all that has supported our learning and growth. "I love you" sends out love to all that is—to ourselves, to others . . . to the world. Sit with these four phrases and wish them to the person or event in your heart that you are having a hard time letting go of or processing. As we grow and expand, soul-work becomes much like cleaning an office or home space. Mental "files" are perused through and examined. Some bring about love, happiness, and joy—so they are shined up and kept for further use. Some are no longer suitable for the current operation, and all is made better, more refined, by replacing, repairing, or altogether tossing them out. Change is inevitable. The willingness to lean into change, based on what *feels* right and best, continually results in moving toward a more fulfilled and aligned version of *being*.

The Energetics of Change

> *"The universe is full of magical things patiently waiting for our wits to grow sharper."*
>
> —Eden Phillpots, author and poet

The study of energy movement fascinates me. Energy cannot be created or destroyed—it is perpetual and can only change form. To change form, energy must be in motion, and all energy follows the basic laws of movement. Movement is vibration, and according to the Law of Vibration, nothing rests. Everything is in a constant state of moving—of vibrating. The Law of Vibration, along with the Law of Polarity (everything is dual) and the Law of Attraction (like attracts like), all work together to help shape our life experience through the balancing out and movement of energy. The Law of Vibration makes sure that nothing ever stays still. The Law of Polarity is at play in the old adage "When one door closes, another one opens," and then through the Law of Attraction, more of whatever we're focusing on strolls right in. Questioning these laws of energetic movement is easy to do—we can't necessarily see them in the palpable ways that some of us need for belief. How much of a role do they really play in the creation of our lives? How much is happening outside of orderly goings-on? Do any of us, while here, have concrete, immobile answers to these questions? I certainly don't.

The Law of Polarity describes everything as being dual. For movement to occur, there must be a positive and negative pole. Another way to explain this duality is that there are two opposite places on the same spectrum, and one cannot exist without the potential for the other. For example, there can't be bad without the potential for good. Hot and cold are two opposite extremes, as well as joy and sadness, fear and courage, yes and no, light and dark. If we look at a situation and see negative, we can also look at it and see positive. These are all varying degrees of the same thing. The place or degree at which something exists can shift by focusing on a different place on the continuum.

The Law of Attraction simply says that like attracts like. We are constantly emitting energy, and this energy pulls similar energy toward it. We, in our most basic form, exist as a vibration. The smallest particles known to man are vibrations. Thoughts are vibrations. Words are vibrations. Sounds are vibrations. Light is a vibration. Even the solid things surrounding us, such as this book, are moving energy. Our amazing planet and everything, seen or unseen, on or within, is a vibrating mass of atoms and subatomic particles. Our collective vibrating energetic masses overlap, interact, and harmonize all day, every day. What we think, what we feel, what we intend, what we desire: these all add to what is on the move within and around us. As we are made of and connected to creative Source Energy, what exists around us has (at least in part) been coming through us. Our life is influenced by the bulk of our thoughts and feelings—the thoughts and feelings that we routinely focus on.

Whether, intentionally, unintentionally, we believe that we're acting alone or we have the universe working alongside us, it is difficult to deny that we are playing some kind of role in creating what our lives look like. And regardless of our personal ideas and what we see as true or accurate, focusing on the goodness in our lives just feels . . . good. So, science and absolutes aside, immersing ourselves in the vision of what we want, what inspires us, what feeds us, and what we find beautiful and uplifting is a helpful place in which to be if our goal is to feel better.

Beyond Thinking to Just Being

The space of pure *being* and *allowing* can also support a lot of positive change. When we notice negative thoughts surfacing—and they, of course, will—there is nothing wrong with sitting with them for a stretch—accepting and embracing them as something to be present with, in an unconditionally tolerant and judgment-free way. Learning from and transforming any troubles that may arise along our path is best accomplished through not only an awareness that they exist, but an understanding that they just might exist for a reason. We are spiritual beings enjoying a human, earthly experience. Through allowing ourselves to experience it all, as it is, and allowing ourselves to *be*, in all the various ways that we are—while learning to embrace anything that makes us feel alive—we allow our path to unfold in a way that honors our spirit *and* our human selves.

Daily Affirmations

Learning to think and speak about the vision of your life in a *present, positive* way can be a worthwhile retraining of the mind. Doing so might help to push the vision of your ideal life forward. Take notice of any moments during which you're focusing on negative feelings or statements and think about how you might be able to reframe them. If you frequently observe and speak about how you feel a certain undesirable way, you might increasingly recognize and resonate with things and experiences that you believe are contributing to this way of feeling. If, instead, you begin to focus on and acknowledge the things and experiences that support an improved outlook, you might be surprised by the way you're more readily able to spot out and let in more moments and experiences that warm your heart and make you smile. For example, if you're constantly monitoring how difficult your relationship with your partner is and you notice and identify more and more with challenging moments, your experience starts to sync up with your focus. Shifting your attention to the love that flows between the two of you, the fun that you have, and your thankfulness for the open, honest relationship that you both get to be a part of can begin to redirect the experience.

Continually focus on feeling into and making positive statements about how you wish your life to be. The world around you, curious and engaged, will turn to notice what you're paying attention to. If there's enough interest and excitement, it might be quick to drop whatever is lacking importance or enthusiasm to come along for the ride. Try to feel, think, and speak about your vision in the present tense (I am, I have, etc.) as if it already exists.

Not on board with the "law of attraction" stuff? Does all of this have you rolling your eyes and wanting to make jokes about turning the nearest pumpkin into a coach by focusing on it long enough? If you're thinking that everybody just needs to put the cap back on the fairy dust and take a few steps back, then I invite you to think about all of this in a more down-to-earth sort of way: focusing on the things that we want for this life is a psychologically sound practice that has the very real capability to move just enough negative dialogue out of the way to make room for something a little better . . . and then a little better . . . and then . . . you get the idea.

You can use the affirmations below for a daily practice, or you can create an entirely new list to better fit you and your life. Take a few minutes, each day, to sit quietly and go through the list, being with each affirmation, or vision, as if it were strong and current—as if it were already established in your life . . . fairy dust optional.

I begin my day in the space of joy and gratitude . . .
and the knowing that all is as it should be.
***

I am whole, healthy, and complete.
***

I am connected to all that is around me.
***

Everything I need is within me.
***

I enjoy the most fulfilling and love-filled relationships.
***

I love who I am and all that I do.
***

All is well.

-Creating Change-

- Become aware of your routine thoughts and how they affect the way you feel.

- Try to let go of thoughts about the past and/or how the future might play out to focus more on the present moment.

- Forgive. Make a list of the people and/or life events in relation to whom/which you carry around negativity and practice Ho'oponopono until you feel this energetic weight being lifted and transformed.

- Take time, each day, to focus on retraining undesirable thoughts through focusing on positive affirmations.

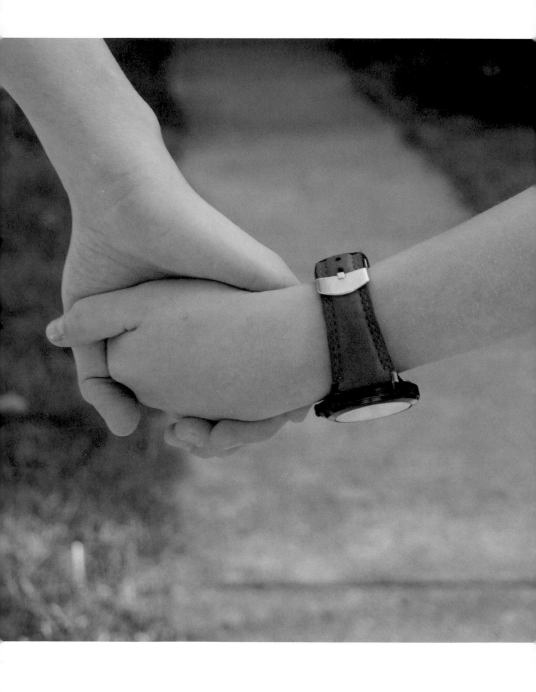

7

I Am Connected (Unity)

"When we try to pick out anything by itself, we find that it is bound fast by a thousand invisible cords that cannot be broken to everything in the universe."

—John Muir, naturalist and author

To Others

Many soul-fulfilling roads lead to, or at least have a lot of memorable sojourns around, connection. It might be one of the larger reasons we are here—and one of the larger instigators of change. It shines big light on purpose and meaning in our lives and presents us with challenges through which we learn and grow. It doesn't matter if we're talking with people who work in biology, psychology, sociology, or medical science: what people in all fields are increasingly grasping is that connection—the ability to feel affiliated, aligned, and united—is an essential component to the design of a physical life that feels significant and satisfying.

We all occasionally encounter core-stirring incidents—situations during which we are faced with change without feeling as though we chose the change. Sometimes we might sense a higher purpose of unexpected events or situations and, as a result, feel sound and whole while anticipating a tweaked reality that is often slightly, if not greatly, better than the present one. Other events might shift our energy and overall sense of safety so quickly that it takes a few sleepless nights and distracted days to fall back into the comfortable, cradled feeling of being safe and where we need to be—emotionally and directionally. During these weightier life moments, it might seem almost as essential as breathing to connect with a couple of really close friends to regain a certain sense of balance. Sharing with those we love and resonate with during any situation that leaves the body and mind asking the questions "What just happened?" and "Where do I go from here?"—those who embody similar energies, mindsets, goals, ideas, beliefs, and humor and/or who are in similar situations—can be soothing and powerful.

We no longer live in true tribal communities. Though we may frequently see one another out during the day, most of us retreat to isolated homes for much of our lives. As a community, we are aware that diet and exercise play a role in health, but it's increasingly difficult for our culture to deny that seclusion weighs in when it comes to how long and how well we are living. The list of hardships that relate to loneliness—lacking deep and meaningful connections with other people—is lengthy and inclusive. Several studies have found that those who are fully devoted to being a stable, steady part of other people's lives—whether the connections be romantic, friendly, or familial in nature—tend to outlive those who are not. Of course, the benefits that arise from the sense of love and connection that committed relationships often embody are not exclusive to those who are legally married, but it's still notable that insurance companies recognize marital status as one of the top indicators of how long a person is likely to live.

Entrainment

Our bodies naturally sync up with the energetic rhythms and pulses around us through a physics principle called entrainment. Entrainment was identified by a Dutch Physicist and Scientist name Christian Huygens in 1665. Huygens found that when he placed two pendulum clocks on a wall near each other and swung the pendulums at different rates, they would eventually sync up and swing at the exact same rate. Whether in a controlled environment or out in nature, there is a tendency for two oscillating bodies to synchronize and vibrate in harmony. The weaker of the two oscillating bodies will adjust to the vibration of the stronger one. Examples of entrainment can be seen mechanically, like the two clock pendulums swinging in unison, or biologically, like when women who spend a lot of time together find that their menstrual cycles begin to sync up. We've all experienced emotional entrainment, like when we walk into a room full of people who are sad and immediately feel the heaviness, or who are happy and laughing and feel the mood quickly lighten. Entrainment can also be seen in the medical community, like when a transplant patient receives a new organ that must entrain to their body in order to be effective.

Entrainment is often at play when it comes to healing. While practicing various energetic healing techniques, many healers are not only acting as a conduit for life force energy, but also focusing on holding a vibration that is powerful enough to be helpful and supportive to another being while sharing healing space. The downside to entrainment is that our body can adjust to the vibration of those who are routinely unhappy or negative. This sprinkles a little bit of science on the saying "choose your friends wisely." Focusing on connections with those who are uplifting is an important part of supporting our own vibrational wellness.

Touch ("The Original Contact High")

"Touch is the central medium in which the goodness of one individual can spread to another. Touch is the original contact high."
—*Dacher Keltner, professor*

We (like all mammals) can live without sight, sound, taste, or our sense of smell, but we cannot function well without touch. There have been plenty of experiments and experiences, throughout our history, that have pointed toward the lifelong effects that warmhearted connection has on the complex network of genetic, neurological, hormonal, and a likely unidentifiable number more of happenings that shape and mold our social behavior and mental/emotional well-being. Research has shown that a mother's nurturing ways can forecast a variety of future behavior. They can predict how well a child does on cognitive tests, how they interact with other kids, and how well they cope with stress. When touch is openly received, the body's vagus nerve carries a feel-good signal to the mood-managing areas of the brain. Activating parts of the brain and releasing hormones, touch can lower blood pressure, heart rate, and cortisol levels.

A good hug, alone—meaning one that is heartfelt and lasts for at least twenty seconds—is right up there with the very best medicines. In our circles of friends and family, hugs quickly and effectively communicate our love and a sense of comfort and presence. I never thought about any measurable effects of hugging until I crossed paths with a study that indicated a significant decrease in stress and increase in immunity in participants who received frequent hugs and felt a greater sense of social support. Experts attribute the stress-reducing, immunity-boosting benefits of hugging to the release of oxytocin—also known as the "love drug"—which lifts levels of feel-good hormones and calms the nervous system. An increase in oxytocin lowers both blood pressure and cortisol (stress hormone) levels. It's often fun (to me, anyway) when science steps in and lays out a story in the quantitative way that it can, but of course we don't need to dive into studies to understand and appreciate the ability that touch has to make us feel happier and more relaxed. We all know that closeness feels good. We know this beyond designs and charts and numbers and calculated outcomes. We live in a society that increasingly shies away from opportunities to connect skin-to-skin, and, while the reasons for this avoidance are understandable, what will the effects be? Are we already seeing them? While it's becoming the accepted norm in our public institutions, I hope that we don't shy away from ongoing, genuine affection within our circles of family and friends. Life and living can be full of tense, hurried moments, but taking the time to pull our partners, our kids, our dear friends close—to hug them, kiss them, tell them that they are loved over and over—is important. These connections are alive with lasting goodness.

Togetherness (Where We Find Home)

"Where we love is home, home that our feet may leave, but not our hearts."

—*Oliver Wendell Holmes Sr., physician and poet*

This morning, while lying in bed, quietly taking in the rhythmic breathing of my children sleeping nearby, I'm reflecting on a stretch of time—not long ago—when there was rarely a moment without one, or both, of these beautiful beings against me; my arms nearly always full with their soft, bare skin; their milky scent after being nourished and nurtured from my heart space; their warm and embraced presence in the bed next to me, during the nighttime hours. I occasionally miss these past moments now as much as I sometimes missed these reflective spaces of stillness and silence then. Both then and now, so much of my time and attention was and is focused upon guarding, supporting, and inspiring the graceful journeys of these sweet souls.

Growing up, I really only knew one home. Our home was surrounded by woods. It was the kind of place that was so dense with magic that if I stilled myself long enough to really focus, I felt certain that I would feel and see things that would raise brows if later spoken about around the dinner table. It was a bright, starry, pine-scented, reliable, and trustworthy place—an area that felt good to connect with and explore. My parents still live there. When I visit, I sleep in the same bedroom that witnessed an incredible amount of growth and change throughout my childhood and teenage years. While wooded visits are not the length or the depth that they once were, amidst more rushed-feeling and shorter stays these days, I love that I can still connect with this space. It feels good to occasionally check in with it; to see and feel the ways that it, too, has expanded and transformed.

After moving away from the home that I grew up in, the routine of moving every year or two commenced without much thought or planning. I enjoy new places, new surroundings, new neighbors, and new paths. It wasn't until after college that I struggled with feeling homesick for a stretch of about three years. Often interesting to me, however, was that the intense longing that I felt was never for my childhood home. Though I didn't realize it at that time, the place that I missed didn't feel as though it were a physical location. I missed a much larger, more expansive place—a collective of beings, of presence, of experience. After our kids joined us, it felt more important to cultivate a space that they could spend many years living in and loving. Deciding to commit to one home has felt right—yet every year, like clockwork, I feel a familiar urge to pack my bags and switch things up. While I really appreciate my childhood home, my idea of "home" and my perceived need to commit to one home has shifted much over the past few years. It has taken a little while to appreciate that home is not always a place with an address. It can be a place that exists, regardless of physical locale, deep within us—always ready and accessible—a connection to the people we love, one that moves and breathes far beyond the boundaries of this earthly life.

Shifting my focus back to my sleeping children, I am reminded that the foundational elements of our lives really don't change much at all. It is in the love that flows among us and the pure perfection of our togetherness where we feel whole—where we find home.

Unfearfully and Wonderfully Present

Earl and Irene were an older couple who attended the church in which I spent Sunday mornings as a child. Earl had the kind of animated sense of humor that, years later, I can still vividly recall. He was the "mint man"—he always divvied out mints from a roll (or likely several) that he kept in his pocket. Irene was equally cheerful. After I was graduated from high school, they stopped by our home, and Irene excitedly handed me a graduation gift. It was a book called *Fearfully and Wonderfully Made*. I remember her telling me about how much she enjoyed it and that she wanted to share it—that she was looking forward to hearing my thoughts about it.

That was over two decades ago.

There isn't much that I would consider doing differently, if I could go back and do anything over. I occasionally think about Irene and this book that she shared with me, however, and imagine having read it sooner. Maybe I would have made a pot of tea and invited her over to talk about it after. I still have the book, but it's too late for that chat, alongside tea, with Irene. Maybe it wasn't even that important to her, but it occasionally surfaces and serves as a reminder, in my life, to be present with the souls I get to cross paths with—to take the time to really see, hear, and be with people, to support their interests, listen to their stories . . . to show up, over and over again.

When we're present, we're not thinking about the past, worrying about the future, or swept up in a sea of distractions. We're tuned in to our surroundings, to whomever we are with, to whatever is happening in this moment. There's a lot going on within the busyness of our lives. It can be a struggle to allow a relaxed focus on the current moment, and, yeah, sometimes it's a whole lot of fun to replay meaningful moments or to dream about the future, but there's big fulfillment, too, in opening our eyes to what is here—even if it's messy and chaotic—and saying, "Hey there. I see you."

To My True Self

Few things push us to learn and to grow as far and as deeply as an intimate relationship. And few of us, within our relationships, have experienced nonstop smooth sailing. When we so closely interlace our worlds and lives with those of another, things are going to crop up that we have to deal with to continue feeding the connection in a way that the connection continues feeding us. Many of us occasionally blame our partner's actions for the way we are feeling, yet our feeling less-than-good is much more about what we are doing to or creating for ourselves than it ever is truly the result of what somebody else is doing to or creating with us. How we feel, what we think, imagine, and expect affect who we are and the world around us.

Self-understanding is one of the most important subjects to address. When we care about the relationship with ourselves, we have a solid foundation for all other connections in our life. While loyal connections support wellness, it is not fair to entirely depend on any other being to feel a certain way. When we're asking or expecting somebody else to lift us up or to help us feel a certain way, we're asking for something that we can accomplish from and within our own selves. We're stepping away from an empowered place of being able to choose how we feel and which experiences we're drawn to and handing this power over to an individual who does not and will never have creative control over our lives.

Feeling well is our natural state. Resistance to the smooth and open movement of balancing energy affects this feeling of wellness—interfering with the ability of our innately intelligent cells to do what they know to do. Whichever tools we choose to help support the process, wellness takes a stronger hold when we shift our focus away from roadblocks around simply feeling good and more toward the feeling good itself. Feeling good, however, doesn't mean that we ignore or stifle unpleasant feelings as they arise within us. All of us, even those who appear to be experts at living a joyful and peaceful life, occasionally face times during which painful experiences usher us into quiet reflection. But these experiences also push us into the space of change—into the space of supporting something different to take form—and often something better. When we do the work of becoming intimate with our true selves and allowing the things that are no longer right for our lives to move out and away, we are also allowing wellness to sweep in, enliven, and uplift.

To Our Earth

Sliding off our shoes and allowing our bare skin to directly connect with the ground is one easy and effortless way to help support the harmonic-with-nature design of our bodies. Being barefoot easily conjures up the feelings of freedom, peace, and simplicity. What is often the norm for young children playing outside seems to dissipate as we begin to interact with the more rushed and routine-centered world that envelops us as we become older.

I've always enjoyed being barefoot outdoors. During my college years, friends would gently tease me about my habit of sliding off my shoes so my bare feet touched the ground the second class was over. Walking home barefoot was a true delight—one that I felt intuitively connected to and instantly at ease with then but wouldn't be able to transmit into words until later. Fast-forward a few years, load up on more responsibilities, and load down on time spent outdoors (sans shoes). For those who are energetically sensitive, this combination can feel really frenetic. I began thinking about the differences in the energetic frequencies outside, emanating directly from the Earth, versus the frequencies inside, emanating from a typical home's mob of technogadgetry, many years before I became motivated and serious enough to dig a little deeper. The moment I became interested in better understanding the science of it all, doors began to open and information became available in the way that it often does when we're ready to receive it.

In the same way that modern buildings and appliances are "grounded," placing our bare skin directly on the Earth physically "grounds" us. This grounding prevents any potential interference that may occur as a result of electrical buildup. While the practice of "grounding" is standard in the care and maintenance of current construction, few of us routinely apply this understanding to our own bodies. We have been blocking the current from the Earth for years, the same current, or flow, that we're designed to be connected with twenty-four hours a day. Most of us spend much of the day in our homes or an office space, and, when we're outdoors, we wear shoes and often walk on asphalt. We move through each day never discharging the free radicals imperceptibly reverberating around us.

Negative Ions, Positive Balance

The Earth is a limitless source of free electrons that stream into the body when it is grounded. This infusion of negative ions from the Earth into the body and the discharge of positive ions from the body into the Earth play a role in feeling well. An excess of positive ions in the body is associated with disorder and degeneration. Negative ions are associated with vitality, good health, and healing. The more time that we spend grounded, the less inflammation our bodies are likely to experience, resulting in improved overall health and a sense of calmness, clarity, and vitality.

Jumping into a body of water or simply touching the Earth with bare feet starts the process of these negative ions cascading up through our body, clearing out positive ions, and restoring balance and a rich overtone of tranquility to our entire system—including our muscles, tissues, bones, and brain pathways. The benefits are almost so easy that they can be readily dismissed by those looking for a more complex path to a better state of health and wholeness. There's an abundance of research now underway, and easy to find in books, online, or through the experiences of others, showing that the process of grounding or connecting with the Earth holds collective and diverse benefits for both the physical body as well as mental and emotional harmony.

Ways to Connect

The most direct and fun way to ground is to simply take off our shoes and socks and walk barefoot outside. We are "grounded" when we are touching the ground, yet whatever is in contact needs to be conductive. There needs to be an electrical connection to the Earth. Rubber, for example, is a barrier to electrical impulses coming up through the Earth. The soles on shoes, then, pose a concern, as most of us wear them all day long. While there are special grounding shoes, which insert conductive material into the soles of the shoe, 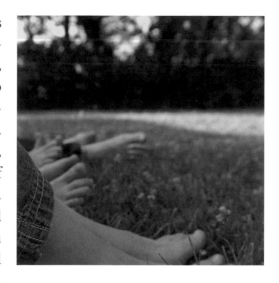 and grounding sheets and bed pads that are now available, which plug into the grounding system of a house for a constant connection, the most effective and appreciably relaxing way of connecting is to directly touch the Earth. When we walk barefoot on the soil or on the beach, we are grounded. When we're swimming, we are grounded. Splashing through a puddle barefoot—grounded. Touching a tree—grounded. Seawater is a great conductor, so walking along the beach and swimming are excellent choices for a strong connection. The conductive choices slim down for those who live in the city, surrounded by asphalt and concrete, yet are still available. Some newer cement may contain polymers that act as an insulator or may be sealed, cutting off its conductive abilities, but most cement, especially older concrete, is grounded. Asphalt, due to its petrochemical content, is not conductive. Even in the city, however, there are patches of grass, gardens, and parks that provide a space to slip off one's shoes.

Spending time in direct connection with the Earth each day may be as fundamental as clean air, water, sunlight, and nutrients. All it requires is that we take the time to get our feet a little dirty, feel the grass between our toes, hang our legs into a river or stream, jump into a lake, breathe deeply, and experience the powerfully effective healing nature of our planet.

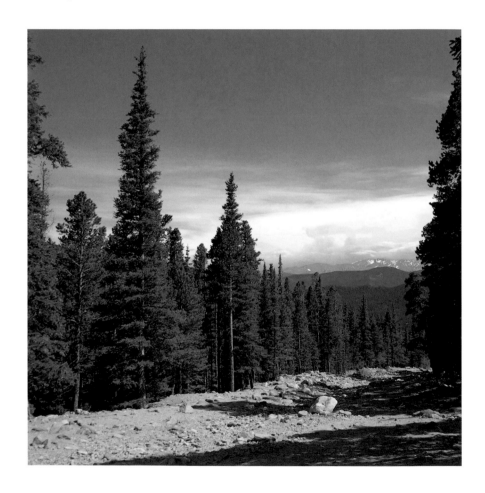

–Creating Change–

- Make time for meaningful connection with those who uplift you. Amidst the busyness of everyday life, try to keep spending quality time with others near the top of your priority list. Schedule a weekly or monthly visit with a group of good friends or plan a date night with your partner.

- Work in some routine quiet time for yourself, too. Consistently tune in to your own body and being, cultivating an inner awareness and sense of safety, regardless of what life brings your way.

- Whether it's a swim or simply slipping off your shoes for a few minutes in the backyard or a nearby park, connect with the Earth, "skin to skin" for a few minutes every day.

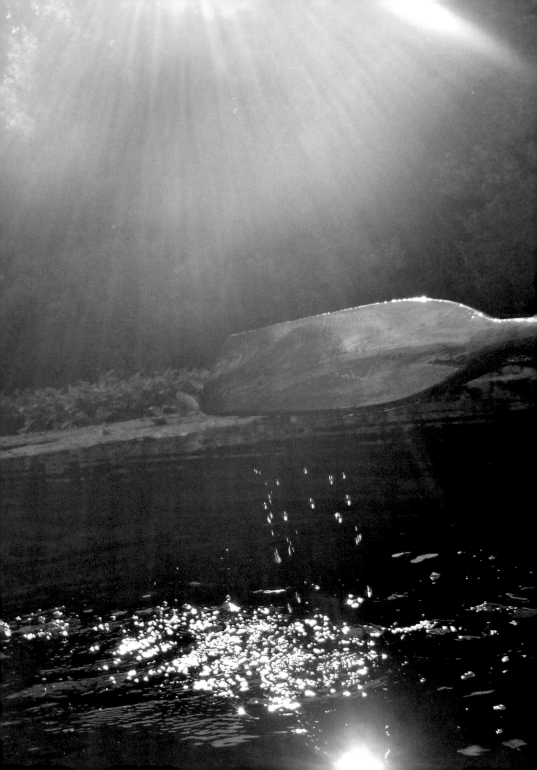

8

I Am Fulfilled (Purpose)

❦

"Three grand essentials to happiness in this life are something to do, something to love, and something to hope for."
—Joseph Addison, poet and playwright

A beautiful friend of mine, who, at the time of this writing, has been living on this planet for eighty-eight years, quickly became one of my favorite people after our paths crossed. She is intelligent, free-spirited, and absolutely thriving. One evening, while out with a local group of friends, I was asked how this older lady manages to maintain such a full and vibrant life. I hadn't given it much thought, yet a reply instantly formed: she has purpose. In her eighty-eighth year, she works full-time from her home. She has a living room full of evidence that her hobbies and interests are continuously expanding. She occasionally jokes around with me about signing up for classes at a local college. She has an active social life and a solid, steady reason to get up out of bed each (very early) morning.

Purpose fills us. It keeps things moving. Meaningful accomplishment feels good. Connection and purpose travel hand in hand. When I want a convincing source of insight and guidance, I often find myself taking a look at various groups of our world's longest-lived people. A few of my favorite books are ones that offer inspiring accounts of extraordinary people living lively, happy lives in some of the most remote parts of this planet. Stories about their ways of living never offer a magic longevity pill or potion. They hold no hidden "one-shot" secrets to health or happiness. Instead, these writings often reveal tales of folks who lend weight to timeless health-supporting routines and perspectives—life recipes that can't be brewed up in any laboratory. They describe people who are firmly woven into tight social fabrics of balanced give-and-take networks and connections, with elders who wake up each morning with a long list of responsibilities. Their lives are rich with purpose and belonging. They feel that their life is part of a larger plan. They are guided by their spiritual values. They are mindfully active and maintain strong cardiovascular and immune systems well into their older years. These people gift to the world a message of encouragement to embrace meaning and connection as a routine way of life.

Fear

"When I dare to be powerful, to use my strength in the service of my vision, then it becomes less and less important whether I am afraid."

—Audre Lorde, writer and civil rights activist

Some children are afraid of the dark. The darkness is a mystery. It is an unknown space, allowing the imagination to create wild scenarios and "what-if" situations. A simple way for a parent to address this fear is to turn on the light, allowing their child to see that whatever was being created in their mind only seconds earlier is not the reality that surrounds them. Most children outgrow a fear of the dark as they consistently allow enough light in to be able to see the truth around them. As adults, life situations can have similarities to this common childhood fear. Most of us have experienced stumbling around in the unknown, fearful of the obstacles that we've imagined for our lives. While some fears are unique illusions, anchoring us to certain places, people, or routines that might not be allowing the freedom that we need to expand, others are natural and innate; they are present with good reason. They keep us from picking up poisonous snakes or walking too far out into the ocean. There are these two sides of fear, two ways of seeing our hesitations that affect the way we negotiate our lives around them.

Each day, we have the opportunity to take a look at any challenges in our lives—to assess why they are present and how they might be helping or holding us back. When they become apparent, we can choose to release negative illusions and embrace light-filled and positive visions and expectations. Understanding that we are here to broaden our lives through *all* experiences supports growth toward appreciating that all is here and now to guide us in this journey. Regardless of how or where we feel that our hesitations are moving us, the further we step back and the larger we allow the picture around us to appear, the smaller and more irrelevant these things— these fears—become. The more we widen the frame, the clearer it becomes that nothing is really as it seems in this physical reality. And if we go the other way, focusing in on the smallest of matter around us, it's just as easy for things to lose their recognizable form. None of the things we see—this book, our clothing, our own hands—are what they seem to be as we look at them right now. If we were able to look deeper, to see into and beyond the structures that make up our physical world, we would see both an intricate and chaotic dance of parts and particles working together to form what we see as the whole of things. Everything surrounding us is constantly fluctuating and in motion, with an appearance that can change depending on how closely we're looking. If we could see the orchestration of things in their most expansive and encompassing form, as well as their most elemental form, we might find ourselves too enchanted and full of wonder to be fearful about the "between"—the not quite this and not really that—that we often see through our human lens.

Passion

> "When you follow your bliss . . . doors will open where you would not have thought there would be doors, and where there wouldn't be a door for anyone else."
> —Joseph Campbell, author and professor

Passion also shares a strong connection with purpose. We all have a deep-seated desire to live a life that is exciting, fulfilling, and fun. We want to wake up in the morning feeling eager to do the things that we have chosen to do. We want to fall asleep at night feeling as though we're accomplishing our goals and making valuable contributions to our world. We each have a special fusion of things to offer that nobody else can offer or give in quite the same way. While our stories may overlap a little or a lot, we all are traveling on a one-of-a-kind path, with one-of-a-kind stops along the way. Arising from our heart-space, our passions are like little clues constantly pointing us in the direction of our best-fit route, lighting an inner fire. This flame incites motion and progress, continually connecting us with more of what we love, with what we're wildly interested in, with our larger life plan. Paying attention to what keeps this inner warmth and light illuminated guides us in cultivating a purpose-packed life. In the space of unrelenting enthusiasm, dreams come alive and meaning flourishes.

Creating a Vision Wish List

Going back to one of the first sentences of this book: What would your life look like if you could create it in a way that makes you feel most happy and whole? When we're clear about the things and ways of living that make us feel happy and whole, these things and ways find a way to show up. But what if we're not clear? We're always in the process of getting to know ourselves better, and, sometimes, the things that we're most drawn to aren't always obvious. During college, I changed my major a few times and, by the final landing, *still* wasn't certain that I had found my way to some big purpose in my life. Here's a really simple way to help clarify this question: Sit down in a cozy, clutter-free space with a pen and a piece of paper. Without much thought (without coming up with reasons and obstacles that could keep you from what you really want), start making a list of things that you would love to do. Begin each sentence with:

When I am most happy and whole, I am _____.

You might jot down things like: "living in a beautiful home with an ocean view," "enjoying a committed and loving relationship," "working with a team of fun and supportive people who share a similar vision," etc. Write down whatever you want, but try keep your vision wishes under twenty. When you feel finished, take a break—maybe only a few minutes, maybe a few days. When you're ready to revisit the list, read through each wish and notice how it makes you feel. Begin crossing off sentences that make you feel less excited. Once you've narrowed it down to only a handful of things that you feel the most excited about, and you're more clear about what your passions are and what makes you feel most happy, it's time to bring in elements from Chapter 6 (p. 75) and give attention to these passions and desires.

Vision Cards

Thanks to the many books and sources of information about this subject, many of us are familiar with vision boards. Vision boards are a creative way of developing clarity around how we want to live and giving attention to these ways of life. I loved the idea of vision boards when I first read about them many years ago but instead like to create vision cards. Vision cards are a simplified version of a larger board. On an index card, write, "I am so happy and grateful," and then complete the sentence with a situation or way of life that makes you feel excited, content, happy, and grateful. Unlike vision boards, vision cards are portable and can be pocketed or placed anywhere you're likely to see them several times a day. Our minds are like computers—and our lives are influenced by whatever we are constantly inputting. A lot of people spend time attending to what they lack or don't want in their lives. When we spend time attending to what we *do* want, the world starts to reorganize around this focus. Vision cards arc an casy way to shift our attention.

Courage

> "*You know, sometimes all you need is twenty seconds of insane courage. Just literally twenty seconds of just embarrassing bravery. And I promise you, something great will come of it.*"
>
> —Benjamin Mee, author

During my first year of college, I was eating in the cafeteria one afternoon when this guy strolled up to where I was sitting. He introduced himself and asked for my phone number. He claimed that his friends had dared him to walk over, cleverly letting me know that it was going to be extra embarrassing if he returned to them empty-handed. A quick glance across the room, to spot a group of lads attentively smiling and watching, confirmed his tale. At first, I remember thinking that it was an odd, slightly immature move, but after a few minutes of witty banter between the two of us, I gave him my number—my *real* number. He became one of my favorite friends that year. Decades later, we still talk. As I think back, quite a few of my favorite friendships have been cultivated after only a few seconds of "embarrassing bravery." These friends, with little to no warning, wowed me with their ability to say, "Yes! Yes, this!" As a naturally playful soul, maybe I was enchanted by the inherent lighthearted nature of these few—or maybe I was drawn to their fearlessness as chances were scooped up while thought was temporarily suspended. Vulnerability, spontaneity, and spirited confidence are all eternally attractive qualities in my world. Whatever it was or is that instantly made our connections a lasting "yes," I sometimes miss it in what often feels like a less risky world these days.

As time passes and responsibilities add up, many of us feel less connected to the unrefined magic within and around us that seems to stir up more passion and adventure than our more calculated, careful actions and decisions. Of course, there are good places and spaces for thorough thoughtfulness, but imagine the potential in allowing an occasional ration of "insane courage" and "embarrassing bravery" to flood the various areas and dynamics of our lives. Stagnant careers could be rerouted, relationships ignited, love deepened, souls enlivened, experiences stumbled upon that might not ever have come our way had we not instantaneously dared them to step closer. Do I have the courage to live beyond the limits I have imagined for myself? This is a question that I hope encourages each of us to, at least occasionally, step out beyond what feels comfortable and safe.

Who Are You to Play Small?

"Our deepest fear is not that we are inadequate. Our deepest fear is that we are powerful beyond measure. It is our light, not our darkness, that most frightens us. We ask ourselves, who am I to be brilliant, gorgeous, talented, and fabulous? Actually, who are you not to be? You are a child of God. Your playing small does not serve the world. There's nothing enlightened about shrinking so that other people won't feel insecure around you. We are all meant to shine, as children do. We were born to make manifest the glory of God that is within us. It's not just in some of us; it's in everyone. And as we let our own light shine, we unconsciously

*give other people permission to do the same. As we're liberated
from our own fear, our presence automatically liberates others."*
                                    —Marianne Williamson, author

The moment I decided to walk away from a career that I had spent
years preparing for felt like neither a moment of insane courage nor
one of embarrassing bravery. I was scared. I didn't have a plan B.
I remember sitting on the couch one day after turning in my resignation letter, yet still having a few more weeks left of the school
year, with a notebook and a pen. I didn't make the sort of list that is
suggested above—because I knew what I wanted to do. I wanted to
build a career doing something that every part of my being instantly
recognized as a "yes!" I wanted to write. I began sketching out a loose
plan about how I was going to step into the writing scene beyond
schoolwork or journal lines. It was messy and heavy with uncer-
tainty . . . and slowly my mind started presenting all sorts of reasons
and obstacles that could keep me from turning this thing that I love
into a career. I knew that it would take a lot of work. I questioned my
commitment. I asked the living-room air around me, "What am I
going to write about that others would even want to read?"

And then a moment arrived—a clear and beautiful juncture that
has me teary-eyed all over again as I type. In this moment, I either
heard or strongly imagined someone say to me, "Who are you to play
small?" *Holy shit.* What a profound question—one that I didn't have an
answer to. Years later, I came across the quote above. Every time I read
it, I am reminded of this moment and the big potential that is within
each of us. I pass this question along to you, with hopes that it will surface in your mind from time to time, reminding you of your unique
gifts and your courageous capability: Who are you to play small?

Authenticity

"The privilege of a lifetime is being who you are."
—Joseph Campbell, author and professor

"Real" is a dish that goes well with everything. Appreciating the value in what we have to give to the world around us and allowing our natural character to come through are important elements when it comes to melding our passions and our purpose into a more clarified and cohesive presence. Feeling valuable helps us bring ourselves to the table each and every time. It supports us telling the story of who we are with our *entire being*. It gives us the courage to feel imperfect and to love the lessons that come to us through anything we perceive as failure. We treat ourselves with kindness and compassion and, as a result, treat all others with this same backbone of tenderness. We are surrounded by and accept connection as a backwash of authenticity. We embrace vulnerability. We trust in the inherent beauty of revealing our true selves, the willingness to be the first to tell someone how we feel, to follow our passions without any guarantees, to put everything into a relationship or a decision that feels so right but may be lacking in sense or reason. *We become willing to let go of who we think we should be in order to be who we are!*

Joy

"When you do things from your soul, you feel a river moving in you, a joy."

—Rumi, poet

When we're giving less attention to unnecessary fears, when we're paying attention to the things that we feel most passionate about, when we're facing our dreams and our visions with bravery and courage, and we're greeting all of this with our true, eternal selves, *we feel joyful.* We are deep-steeped in that feel-good energy that arises within us when we are fluidly moving forward, yet content with where we are.

This is joy.

Joy, in many ways, is the ultimate purpose. Feeling joyful lets us know that we are stepping in the right direction, while also acting as a foundational magnet for drawing in more of whatever makes us feel excited and alive. During times of stagnancy, when we feel as though we're not moving anywhere, it becomes difficult to really enjoy the world around us. A connection with our purpose may seem so distant as we struggle to search for something that fills us. Yet when we're checked in with our true selves and we're following the internal guidance that is always leading us forward on our uniquely purposeful path, we know the life-loving energy of joy.

> *"Each person comes into this world with a specific destiny—he has something to fulfill, some message has to be delivered, some work has to be completed. You are not here accidentally—you are here meaningfully. There is a purpose behind you. The whole intends to do something through you."*
>
> —*Osho, spiritual teacher*

-Creating Change-

- Reassess the things that you feel fearful about and determine whether these things are helping or holding you back.

- To help clarify what you're most passionate about and allow these passions to lead the way, make and sort through a vision wish list.

- As a way to help focus on the things and ways of life that you're most drawn to, create vision cards. Toss these cards into a bag to carry with you or place them wherever you're likely to see them several times a day.

- During moments when you may feel less than brave, remember that you're a big and important part of this life. Who are you to play small?

- Support your sense of joy through allowing your true self to come through, brightly influencing the world around you.

9

I Am Whole
(Love)

⇛⇛⇛ ⇜⇜⇜

"Don't move the way fear makes you move.
Move the way love makes you move.
Move the way joy makes you move."

—Osho, spiritual teacher

I am Whole *and* I am Love. Loved, yes . . . but bigger: I *am* Love.
Doesn't this just feel good to say? These words create a wave
of chills that move through my body, carrying with them medicine that is strong and soft and unrivaled. Love is innate and inter-
woven into everyone and everything, and, through it, we relate to all
life. It is the ultimate vibration with which we are naturally aligned.
It is a divine, sacred, magical state—vitally important and powerfully
influential. Love deeply heals. It ushers the world toward wholeness.
Reciprocally, feeling whole—content, connected, complete, full, and
balanced—supports the energy of love within and around our lives.

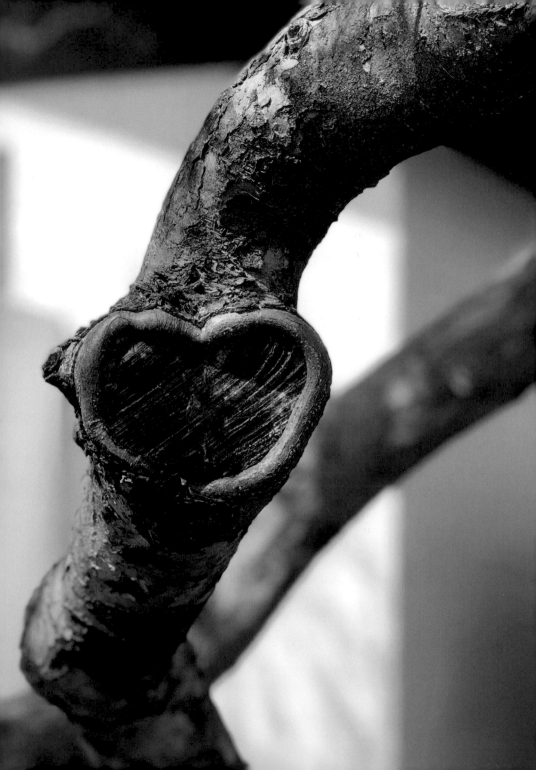

Loving Ourselves

"You cannot get through a single day without having an impact on the world around you. What you do makes a difference, and you have to decide what kind of difference you want to make."
—Jane Goodall, anthropologist

For some, the idea of love begins with an awareness of the feelings of familiarity, safety, and comfort. These feelings have a very real and physical effect on our health. As already mentioned, touch, alone, can have a huge impact on mental and emotional well-being—and can significantly affect biological function, including immune system response. As a person moves on in the evolutionary journey of their soul, love, too, moves beyond the enjoyment of connection or the sense of comfort and safety to embody something much larger. It progressively expands, becoming an all-embracing and circular presence—an expression of joy and happiness emerging from deep within one's self. In its stripped-down essence, love has little to do with any other person or surrounding situation. Love is about coming home to our true self. It is rooted in living from the core, in ways that are in harmony with our being and our planet. When we recognize and allow this alignment, everything around us seems to flow with ease.

The information throughout all of the chapters in this book supports the wellness of our own being. When we're thoughtfully nourishing ourselves, when we're breathing deeply, moving and resting regularly, supporting our body's processes, focusing on uplifting thoughts, and creating lives full of connection and fulfillment, we're directing an incredible amount of encouraging support our way. All of these things nurture our sense of love, and love—as part of all things—nurtures our sense of wholeness. Learning to fully embrace, accept, and unconditionally love who we are forms a foundation for fully loving one another and loving our planet.

Loving One Another

"When the story of these times gets written, we want to say that we did all we could, and it was more than anyone could have imagined."

—*Bono, singer-songwriter*

Settling into feeling a sincere love for all others doesn't mean that we need to strive toward some unreasonable expectation of genuinely enjoying all others. We do not need to admire or applaud the character or the actions of every single person we meet to express and feel unconditional love for them. The contrast on this planet plays a big role in our learning and growth, yet, even amidst aversion, we can remain aware of and further develop an appreciation for all others. We can choose to love them because they share the same energetic space and universal consciousness. Love them for the process that they are bravely going through to learn *here and now*—same as us. Love them because we are connected to them, in a very real sort of way.

Often woven into patterns of feeling anger or dislike is the feeling of judgment: imposing our personal beliefs, ideas, and expectations onto others. Judgment does not change anything in, on, or about the person *being* judged. Instead, it interferes with the harmony and vibration of the one judging. Understanding that we all come through this life collectively, yet with separate missions and purpose, goes a long way when it comes to releasing the desire to want others to learn identical and individually tailored lessons.

Holding on to the idea of absolute truths—to the idea of uniform "rights" and "wrongs"—can be tricky. Maybe the truth is that there are layers and shades of truth. But even if truth is absolute, we are not. We are constantly changing and seeing things differently as we move forward. The moment we see truth as anchored or fixed, we risk closing ourselves off to growth. Most of us have things that we believe to be true right now that we didn't years or maybe even days ago. Truth can incrementally reveal itself. It can unfold in steps—each portion expanding us and preparing us for a larger dose. It asks us to be present and patient. It asks us to allow others to travel at their own pace. It sees us trying to be consistent and instead invites us to just be honest, to be open, to accept any chaos as an opportunity to cultivate clarity.

Maybe you're feeling a bit confused about, overwhelmed by, or resistant to the idea of being connected to everyone and everything. Wherever we each are in this journey is okay. We always have more ahead. The encouragement right now is to acknowledge that we all are here, doing this whole life thing, side by side. Recognizing this togetherness might illuminate a common thread of wanting to bring about both personal and global transformation, and breathe some strength into our collective capacity and capability. And all of this—this capacity, this capability, this change—is hugely supported through the *Love* that we gift to and receive from those around us each day.

Loving Our Planet

"The earth is what we all have in common."
—*Wendell Berry, novelist and environmental activist*

Our time spent here on this planet is short. While how we live for ourselves is impactful, how we live for our planet will have effects that far outweigh and outlast the decisions that we make for our own personal journey. In Chapter 6 (p. 75), we touched upon the ways in which we influence our individual lives. We, combined, hold this same ability to influence our entire world. The more people who are aware of and devoted to the vision of our planet as whole and healthy and who are devoted to the everyday practices that support this vision, the more powerful it becomes and the more it emerges as our reality.

Though my outlook and approach to this issue have slightly morphed over the years, I recall from a young age being concerned about the health and well-being of our natural world. In the past, I've described the way that I feel as though I'm constantly walking out of my front door to find a loved one surrounded by a careless, unaccountable crowd—and I can't break through or do anything to stop the situational momentum. Many nights, while imagining the ways that our world is being forced to change and adapt, I have cried while drifting off to sleep, yet I have always felt hopeful and determined to do something, *anything,* to help make a difference for her and all who depend upon her to survive and thrive. While much of my time and energy has been focused on just our environment, I increasingly recognize and appreciate the strong and undeniable connection between self-love and planetary love. The previous sections come together to effectively care for and support the wholeness of ourselves. Caring for ourselves seamlessly translates into a natural and very innate desire to love and care for our planet. We cannot expect to support our own well-being without also choosing to support the well-being of the place we live. Through holding the vision of our planet as a vibrant, healthy, happy being; taking action and making decisions in our daily lives that reflect an understanding of how deeply connected we are with our Earth; and holding intimate space to connect with her and others in a trusting and faithful way— we'll continue to create big and beautiful change.

Brown Van Simple

"Just as free, free as we'll ever be"

—*Zac Brown Band*

During one unforgettable year, my boyfriend and I enjoyed some amazing road trips in an old brown van that carried him back to school following the long summer break. We drove, stopping anywhere we wished for as long as we wished, taking along only a few articles of clothing, a couple of blankets, pillows, and a one-pan, propane stove. We often made soups and grilled sandwiches on the small stove, and, if we were cooking streetside that night, we ate and laughed with the lively and unexpectedly untroubled homeless people who sometimes joined us. After the night's laughter settled, the conversation felt complete, and our new friends disappeared into the night air, we made love in our Chevy van, and that was all right with us. (This 1973 song tweak seems inescapably fitting.)

We fell asleep happy. When I think about the most free-feeling and inspiring periods of time during my life, the years during which I had very little to keep track of (the days of the old brown van included) immediately surface in my mind. The van didn't last long, but the lingering remembrance of a simpler way of living will stay with me always.

Compared to most of the people we know today, my family has few material things, and simplicity courses through the veins of our daily rituals and creations. But it's not brown van simple. We have a small home to constantly upkeep and an accompanying mortgage to pay off. We have a yard to mow and rake. We have daily commitments that don't always (or even often) support taking off for long stretches of time with little idea or concern about when we will be returning to it all. There is a sense of freedom that travels alongside simplicity—and this unhindered harmony has far-reaching effects.

The Ripple Effect of Simplicity

"Have nothing in your house that you do not know to be useful or believe to be beautiful."
—*William Morris, textile designer and novelist*

Home—noun; the place where one lives permanently. There are many things to think about when it comes to creating a healthy home and living space. Air and water quality; the avoidance of using cleaning and lawn-care chemicals; electrical/energetic interferences; whole, nutrient-rich food availability; and mindfully interacting with our spaces of living and rest are only a handful of considerations. As much as I am interested in creating and supporting a healthy space for my family, I'm just as interested in helping to create and support a healthy global space for all of our families, so when I write "home," I am thinking far beyond the boundaries of each of our earthly spaces. Thinking about it in this way often takes both my mind and my practice beyond what I do for and in our own small living space. The ways in which each of us goes about our everyday lives and interacts with the world around us have a phenomenal impact on the health of our planet and are important components of global transformation. Getting back to a more harmonious way of living with our Earth is a process—as many of us have only known a more modern way of living and have, as a result, stepped away from some of the more foundational, nature-connected ways of living and of loving. There are many daily practices we can focus on with the goal of making an environmental difference. Amidst this list, living a very simple life is something that stands out, over and over again, as a "yes!" Through letting go of the importance of material things, many other, more ecofriendly ways of living are inherently woven into the scene.

What makes a life feel simple and sustainable is a bit different for each of us. For me, simplicity in the ways that I live involves a focus on what feels most foundational and beautiful. It involves stepping away from what is inessential and/or harmful to my personal living space and our planet and leaning toward more time spent with the people I love and the routines and events that feel important and valuable to me. Creating a simple home space, however, isn't always a simple process, especially when others—who are weaving their own unique visions, desires, and ideas into the mix—are living alongside. It is an ongoing practice that becomes an ingrained and instinctive way of life—not something to be completed in an afternoon or weekend. Simplifying our material load starts with identifying what is most important to us—what makes us happy, what fills and sustains, what we "know to be useful" or "believe to be beautiful." Whatever doesn't make the cut receives a nod of gratitude before finding itself on a new path or in a new home. Most important when it comes to reducing the amount of material waste that we collectively generate is to focus on only buying things that we *really* want and/or need—and, even then, being conscientious of what we're investing in. Instead of thinking about price, think about lasting value. Consider how many years an item is going to be used before it finds a spot in a nearby landfill. The drift for many in our current society is to collect and hold onto material belongings as if they both create and define a person. I have really enjoyed the process over the past few years of releasing belongings that I no longer have use for or find simple bliss in keeping around—and, in many ways, allowing more space for freedom and authentic connection.

As important as the tangible components that outline one's living space are the energetic ones. Our home environment affects our presence and thoughts—and our thoughts are, again, influential when it comes to our overall well-being. Our home—whether we imagine it as a physical structure with a street address, as wide-spanning as the entire planet, or just the space of togetherness that was brought up earlier—is not truly a permanent place of residence in this dynamic life and world. What we'll leave behind may feel less important when compared with what we'll take with us from this experience, but for the sake of caring well for her *and* for ourselves while here, the Earth is our home—and it is and will be the home for generations of loved ones following us. Regardless of the specific ways in which each of us chooses to create and maintain structure and sanctity within our living space, remember that the larger goal is to make conscientious and respectful decisions in *all* of the ways that we choose to live our lives—and to cultivate a presence and life practice that fills our signature purposes for being here on this planet.

Every day, I crave loving communion with this planet.
I speak with her.
I listen to her.
I touch her.
I soften against her touch.
I celebrate her.
I hand over my visions and my dreams, and I trust in hers.
I pray for balance and for healing; for her; for us—one and the same.

An Invitation

At some point, throughout each day, I go through a series of affirmations. I focus on the devotion that I feel toward myself, my family, you, your family, and toward our Earth. I focus on the power that is within and around me. I focus on the passions that I am leaning into—and what these passions are bringing through to this world. I discover and feel the peace that comes through allowing these joyful interests to take the lead. I radiate love outward, starting with what's nearest to me: my own body/being, the bodies/beings of my children, my neighbors, my friends, larger and larger—until I feel as though I'm holding the entire planet in my heart/soul-space. It can be challenging to create change that feels as though it's effective beyond our immediate surroundings—that feels as though it will last and give birth to more change. This prayerful routine feels powerful and capable. It is my favorite ritual of the day. It's not a replacement for action—for living in ways that more tangibly support the wellness of life around us—but it builds and instills optimism around both our sense of hope and our ability to achieve clear and consequential revisions. Change seems to arrive more readily in the company of inspiration or encouragement than it does surrounded by doubt or distrust. I invite you to join in this vision and practice—in whatever ways feel good and right to and for you.

When I first began working on this book, my focus was more on each individual who would be reading. When seeing a chapter title, my mind often replaces "I" with "We"—you, everyone, everything, and myself; all one and the same. *We* are whole. Together, *we* have the ability to make a significant and lasting difference. Whatever it is, bring it back to love and watch it transform into something different, something better, something whole.

–Creating Change–

- Feel into your connection with everyone and everything.

- When you feel judgmental, pause to ask how whatever you are questioning might be serving another soul.

- Devote a few minutes, each day, to envisioning our planet as vibrant, healthy, and happy.

- As an effective way to live more harmoniously with the natural world, focus on creating a small and simple living space, containing only things that you love and/or regularly use.

- Be mindful of what you buy. Consider things like whether packaging is recyclable, how long the item will last before it finds its way to a landfill, and, most important, whether it's something that you really want and/or need.

- In the same way that you use affirmations to create change within, use them to send loving, transformative energy outward—helping to support global change.

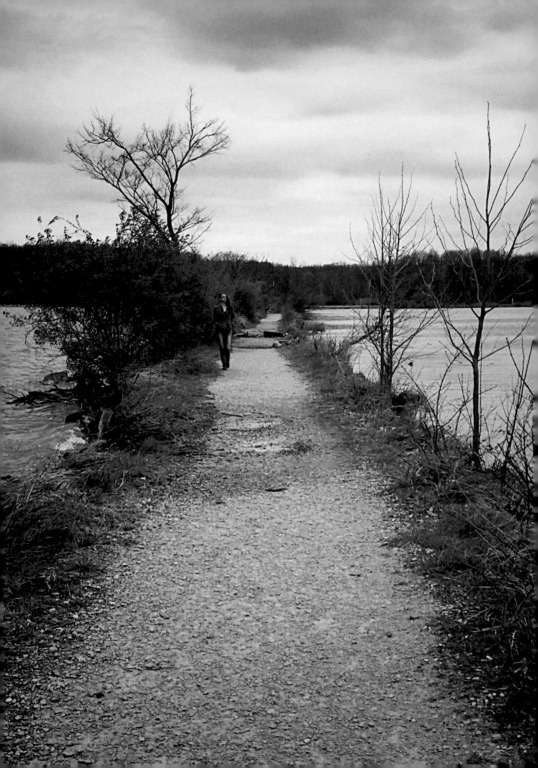

Onward and Upward

"Anything can happen, child. Anything can be."
—Shel Silverstein, writer

The road toward any place is a process; it is a journey—one that is full of reminders, growth, and evolvement. If needed, it might take time for the body to heal, for physiology to shift. Being with and allowing this time is important. Today and tomorrow will never be what yesterday was, nor would we ever truly wish them to be. In the swirl of change, hold strong to the belief that *anything is possible*. The desires or visions that this world inspires within us are ones that we can achieve. There is a force that lives within each of us—an energy, a capability, a competency—that nothing in this world can touch. With our familiarity and trust in this abiding presence arrives the deeper awareness that what we are limited by is greatly influenced by what we *believe* we are limited by. So much starts to shift as we learn to let go of perceived limitations, to live attuned to nature and to our own intuition, and to get cozy with our boundless strength and abilities.

Does trusting in our hopes and dreams mean that we won't encounter rougher moments? Probably not—but walking through the darker events of our lives often leads to a place where a lot of good can be recognized. Discomfort is an amazing teacher—maybe one of the greatest. As a friend and messenger, it insists on being witnessed, acknowledged, and surrendered to. It requires digging down deep, intermingling the light with the dark, and stepping outside of where we were previously comfortable before it's ready to take off. We may not always be able to understand what the world is bringing our way during each moment, and there might be plenty of occasions that have us feeling as though we're not equipped to handle the responsibility of this adventure with grace and wisdom. Crossroads aren't always clean. When we meet up with messy junctures, it's helpful to remember this: We chose this journey. I chose it. *You* chose it.

What I have been grateful to observe, over and over, as others invite me in and open up (and as I further open up to myself and all that is around me) is that big messages, tidy or otherwise, rarely arrive as random experiences. Maybe they're delivered through our truest, highest selves—or through something even larger—always relevant and right on time. Throughout it all, our job is to stay connected to one another, to our natural world, and to the place within us that effortlessly resonates with the Divine and simply *knows*. We are here to learn, to grow, to encourage lives of extraordinary beauty, peace, and joy, and to exhibit deep care for ourselves, our planet, and all other creatures we share it with. This ability, responsibility, and cocreative energy aren't within a few select people; they are *innate within all of us*. We are powerful shape-shifters and healers. The changes that we hope for and envision for ourselves and for our planet are ready—and we are ready to support these changes through seeing them clearly, believing in them, and living in a way that writes them back into the forefront of our everyday being. Sometimes we're guided to search outward for answers and understanding. We are all here, feeling our way around and walking down this path, together—so when help is wanted or needed, please ask for it. There are so many people, around us, ready and willing to offer support and a soft landing. Keep in mind that a healer supports and empowers you to heal yourself. While guidance may be welcomed and divinely orchestrated, we all have the ability to move toward balance. A healer's role is that of a mentor and a conduit. I have studied alongside and learned from some really gifted healers during this life, yet the most powerful and balancing experiences have arisen from a place beyond tool and technique. I am repeatedly awed and humbled by the things that happen when the stars align in an instinctively restorative way—allowing an incomparable moment to emerge and reveal something that is as mysterious as it is magical.

When turning outward doesn't quite fit, try turning inward. Our internal guidance system is an accurate measure of path alignment. We each can readily tap into it during this earthly incarnation. If something feels good and right for our unique life, it is at least worthy of further exploration. Anything that serves to help settle us into our own source-connected core will also help guide us in trustworthy ways.

Outward, inward, and still not feeling as though you're finding what you're looking for? None of us are here with only an earthly compass. Though not always easily apparent, there is a wellspring of beyond-earthly guidance surrounding us. This guidance comes through in many different forms. We are *never* alone. During moments we feel lost or off-track, we can always ask for help navigating and allow ourselves to be open enough to receive direction. And there is prayer, a haven of reliable reassurance. Prayer is not about our words. It is not a fixed routine, or an act that we do without much thought or feeling. Authentic prayer is a conscious connection with God—whatever we imagine the energy of God to be. It is full of intent and faith. It is sincere and honest. It wraps us in warmth, clarity, and peace . . . and it can look and feel different for each of us.

Happiness, wholeness, freedom, joy. All of these sensations are steady delights, emanating from within, that exist when we're aligned with the way in which it's all playing out. And if we're not? In this world that is so full of choices, it's not too difficult to wander away from a path that feels comfortable and easy. Should you find yourself momentarily surrounded by rugged ground, please don't stop holding the vision of what a smooth and enjoyable experience would look like for you— what it would sound like, what it would *feel* like, what it would *be*. Lean into allowing these limitless visions and dreams—the variety of dreams that leave you questioning the world, both tangible and not—that lift and leave you open to recognizing and exploring the path that spiritedly winds through and connects the two. Be willing to reconnect with the inspiration that circulates through and from your own imagination, and to dream in big, bold ways.

Creating the lives that we want feels like an enchanting concoction of science and mystery, and while there will always be more to explore, I've come to understand this:

Whatever it is that you want for your life, want it with all of you. No maybes, no plan Bs or Cs, no only if it's easy or only if you have the resources to start, no playing small, no holding back, no second guessing whether you deserve it or can live up to the dream. None of this. Just ask for it and know that it is coming.

Travel through, as often as you wish, being and breathing with each change-creating truth . . .

I am nourished.

I am relaxed.

I am free.

I am renewed.

I am pure.

I am creative.

I am connected.

I am fulfilled.

I am—We are—whole.

Acknowledgments

A special thanks . . .

To Emory and Evan: I am in awe of you, beautiful souls. Thank you for being here.

To Andy: for your presence, devoted love, and friendship . . . and for the many hours that you've patiently spent listening to me read.

To Cody and my animal friends and teachers: for your unique guidance and wisdom, and your source-connected inspiration to live in the moment. Forever and always, you are a part of me, and I am a part of you. Thank you. I love you.

To Jenny: for unknowingly planting a seed and for a friendship that I deeply treasure.

To Mike: for unexpected accountability.

To Marilyn, Michele, and Lucinda: for your expert guidance during the proposal-writing process.

To Renée: for all of the ways that you inspire goodness and change.

To Nicole: for seeing this, for seeing me, and for the incredible work that you do.

To Haven and Raphael: for your gentle guiding presence during some of my most vulnerable and transitionary moments. I see you. Thank you.

To our planet: for your vast beauty and your steady, sustaining ways.

To my parents and brothers: for a lifetime of togetherness and laughter.

To family and friends: that we get to journey together is one of my greatest joys.

—And—

To God/Source/Spirit: in all beings, places, and things, I see and feel you. Thank you for this.